INTERMITTENT FASTING for Women

OVER 50

THE ULTIMATE GUIDE TO ACCELERATE WEIGHT LOSS, RESET YOUR METABOLISM, INCREASE YOUR ENERGY AND DETOX YOUR BODY

WILLIE GOODING

This page was intentionally left blank

CONTENTS

PREFACE

It can be difficult for women over fifty to maintain a healthy weight and keep up with an energetic lifestyle. That is why this book, Intermittent Fasting for Women over 50, was written with the intention of helping you take control of your health. This book will show you how intermittent fasting can help you lose weight fast and detoxify your body while still eating delicious food!

Intermittent fasting is a dieting method where you fast for 16 hours and eat your meals during the remaining 8 hours. This works due to the way our bodies have evolved to function, by alternating periods of fasting and feasting.

The key to successfully losing weight through intermittent fasting is eating the right foods at the right times. This book will also show you how to get the most out of this diet plan by eliminating processed food and simple sugars from your diet. These detoxifying recipes have been specifically chosen for their ability to help you lose weight.

You will learn various methods for intermittent fasting, including one method where you can eat delicious foods and still lose weight! Using these methods in combination with this easy-to-follow diet plan will make it simple to reap the many benefits of intermittent fasting, while still losing those pesky pounds!

"INTERMITTENT FASTING FOR WOMEN OVER 50: The Ultimate Guide to Accelerate Weight Loss, Reset Your Metabolism, Increase Your Energy and Detox Your Body" is a very helpful resource. It contains invaluable information that is presented in an easy-to-read format. I would certainly recommend it to anyone who needs to lose weight or simply wants to be healthier.

WHO IS THIS BOOK FOR?

This book is for women over the age of 50. This book will discuss intermittent fasting for hormone balancing, weight loss, and improved energy levels. In addition, it is perfect for people with a busy schedule who do not have the time to grocery shop or cook every day. You have gone through menopause and feel that your body has slowed down quite a bit. You find it hard to lose weight and often gain weight easily. You feel that you are not as energetic as you used to be and would like to change that as well. You are worried about your health and want to improve your overall wellness.

If this is, you will want to read this book. You will find all the information that you need to learn how to start intermittent fasting for hormone balancing, weight loss, and increased energy levels. You will also learn how intermittent fasting can help detox your body and reduce any issues with digestion or constipation that you may be struggling with now. This book is intended for women over 50 but is useful for people of all ages. If you are looking for a way to help your body feel happier and healthier, then this book is right for you.

The core part of this book is intermittent fasting and how it can help women over 50 with hormonal balance, weight loss, and enhanced energy levels. The book also discusses detoxification as well as eating plans to get started with intermittent fasting. By implementing the guidelines in this book, you can reduce your risks for various health conditions and improve your mood. You will learn about how intermittent fasting can help you lose weight and boost the fat burning process of your body. You will also learn about how to not only lose weight but keep it off as well.

Introduction

Perhaps you've noticed that the weight is creeping up on you as you approach 50. Maybe your body isn't feeling as good as it once did, and you find that many of the things that used to be effortless are now more difficult. Or maybe you haven't noticed any changes and are just curious about what it could do for you. Your body is changing, whether you like it or not. And while aging will happen whether you want it to or not, there are things that you can do to turn the tide in your favor and make it a whole lot easier for your body to stay healthy and move well. Intermittent fasting is one of those things. You'll get much of the same benefits of going on a restrictive diet by fasting intermittently for 16 hours at night and eating normally during the 8-hour day period when you're awake.

Aging is natural, but it's not supposed to be an inevitable process of degradation. It's your body's natural response to stress. Healthy cells respond to stress by slowing down and reducing their rate of repair and reproduction, so they can have the energy to stay alive. Aging is the opposite of that. Your body uses up all of its resources trying to stay alive, so there are none left over for the cells to stay healthy and keep fighting off free radicals and disease. Intermittent fasting helps your body respond more like a younger person's does, with a healthy balance between damage control and repair work.

It's not just your cells that benefit from intermittent fasting. Your whole body responds more efficiently. The resting metabolic rate, or the energy your body uses to keep itself running while you're at rest, goes up by as much as 15 percent after a few days of intermittent fasting. That means that while you're at rest, you burn about 15 percent more calories than usual. It also means that when you exercise, it will be easier for your body to go right back into fat burning mode after you're done. And there's another bonus—your hunger hormone levels stay lower, so when you are hungry, it's easier to find a healthy snack instead of laying down the chips and salsa or going for something high in saturated fat and calories. The visual changes you start to notice in the mirror and your closet will make your more confident, too.

Fasting for 16 hours won't just help you lose weight; it's also good for your heart. Intermittent fasting tells your body that it's not in starvation mode, which helps lower cholesterol and triglyceride levels. It also lowers blood pressure, so it's easier for your body to stay healthy and look great. You'll feel better overall, so there will be no reason not to exercise more and look better. The right exercise can help you lose weight, but it can also help reduce joint pain and stiffness while boosting energy and mood. It can even improve the quality of sleep you get at night between fasts.

Intermittent fasting has no side effects. There are no pills or procedures to put your body through. You don't need to have any special equipment, either; it's all happening on the inside. It can be hard to believe that something so simple could make such a big difference in your life, but it really does. Most people who try intermittent fasting observe changes in as little as two weeks, and there is no maximum number of days per week you have to fast for it to work.

Fasting = Weight Loss

When your stomach is empty, it only wants the nutrients found in food that passes through it and any extra weight that happens to be hanging around outside of your body will pass through with it. Fasting is a great way to lose weight because it allows your body to eliminate the extra waste that it wouldn't get rid of otherwise.

One reason that people find it so difficult to lose weight is that there's still a lot of glycogen in their cells. Glycogen is the stored form of carbohydrates, and it need to be cleared out before weight loss can be achieved. In fact, studies have shown that roughly five pounds of water weight can be lost when the glycogen is replaced in your system. Losing water weight isn't easy when you're just starting off with fasting, but once the glycogen stores are full again, the body will hold on to any additional water as well. That's why it's so crucial for you to drink plenty of water before beginning a fasting diet plan.

When you take in nothing but water during your fast, you truly put your body into starvation mode. This is because our bodies have evolved to survive, and when calories are scarce, they become very efficient at storing every bit of energy that we consume. A single day without food for an active man could produce up to 3 or 4 pounds (1.4 – 1.8 kg) of weight loss simply because of this biological response to starvation.

Fasting = Healthy Cells

When you fast, your body reduces its energy expenditure and shifts to preserve what's most important to its survival. It stimulates stem cell production and the regeneration of healthy tissue. New healthy cells replace dying or diseased ones, and your organs return to their normal youthful function. This is due to a reduction in free radicals—cellular waste that can lead to damage of the heart tissue.

Your body also stops working so hard to digest food, so it can devote more energy to getting rid of toxins in the body. Fasting also increases the production of human growth hormone, which helps you maintain a healthy metabolism and even build muscle while burning fat. It also improves memory and helps your brain stay sharp. Fasting is a natural way to keep your body looking and feeling younger than its years—and that's something we should all strive for as we get older.

Fasting = Healthier Heart

Your blood pressure is lower on fasting days because your body shifts from glucose (sugar) burning to fat burning mode. This means that the fats circulating in your blood are broken down into ketone bodies that travel through the bloodstream to be used by the tissues as they need energy, rather than staying in circulation where they can cause damage. This is especially good for your heart, since it's likely to be affected by high blood sugar levels.

The fasting cycle also increases the amount of good HDL (the "clean" cholesterol) that's present in the bloodstream while lowering the overall LDL (the "dirty" cholesterol) count. This is an ideal situation if you have been told that you're at risk for heart disease, as your cholesterol levels should be getting healthier and not worse. This may be a direct result of the decrease in triglycerides during your fast as well, which have harmful effects on blood vessels and tend to increase your chances for stroke or heart attack.

Fasting = Increased Energy

When you first begin fasting, you may experience some dizziness or weakness. This is just your body adapting to its new source of energy; once it gets used to it, you will feel stronger than ever before. You will have more physical energy and mental vigor, and since you're not putting any bad nutrients into your body (there's no food to digest), all that energy is going toward fighting disease and repairing damage.

The most noticeable result of fasting is how much more energetic you feel. This is because you are giving your cells a boost of ketones (the type of fat that circulates in your bloodstream when you're burning fat). When there are plenty of these ketones around, the brain doesn't need as much sugar—so it actually slows down the aging process, improves memory, and protects against Alzheimer's Disease.

Intermittent fasting has many health benefits, but the increased energy that you get from it is one of the most noticeable. If you've ever tried to reduce your sugar intake and felt like it made you tired and cranky, then fasting should make you feel considerably better.

The main reason this happens is because of a hormone called ghrelin. Ghrelin stimulates your appetite; when your body doesn't get enough food to produce it, you feel hungry all the time. Conversely, when your body gets used to having all its needs provided for during a fast, it produces less ghrelin with each passing day—which means that by day three or four of a fast, you start feeling less hungry and more energized.

<u>The stages of IF</u>

The stages of intermittent fasting

1. Curiosity

You've heard of this "diet" that people are doing, and you're curious about it. You've always been pretty healthy and pretty fit. What harm can it do to see what all the fuss is about? You've seen pictures of people's before-and-afters, and it looks like they lost a lot of weight in a short time. Maybe you're not overweight, but just want to drop a couple of pounds fast to get that beach bod for the summer. It looks pretty simple. But what happens after you fast? If it makes you feel bad, you can just eat the food your body needs to heal, right? There's no need to subject your body to the stress of starving. Hunger is a big signal that your body is in distress. When you're hungry, your brain sends messages to your stomach and other organs saying "Feed me!", and they do exactly that. When you're fasting, however, this process goes awry because your cells no longer get the message that you're hungry. Your brain says "Hey! I'm ready for food! Feed me!" and hunger is shut down completely as even the desire to eat disappears from the body altogether. This, by the way, is why hunger is signaled less when you're fasting. If you break from a fast, there's no longer hunger to tell the brain that it needs food. Your body needs to start this process all over again if it wants to get full. The first day of fasting will be easy. You'll feel hungry and probably have thoughts of eating in your head, but give in and wait for that "furious" feeling or that "dry mouth" which indicate that hunger has been activated. You can just sip on some water or drink some juice or whatever and suppress those thoughts once your stomach starts rumbling, as we mentioned earlier.

2. Excitement

You've decided that you're not shooting for a bikini body, so you can skip step 1 completely. You're going to try fasting every day or at least for a couple of days. You're not worried about what it feels like, only what it will do to your body in the long run. You might even be reckless and attempt twice-a-day or even three times a day (which we'll talk about later). By now you might have reached that "furious" feeling, but are still unsure whether you should go ahead. You're still technically hungry, which is why all those thoughts are popping into your head.

And then there's the bloating and stuffiness under your tongue that we mentioned earlier. There's also the thing that some people experience called "fasting headaches."

3. Confusion

You're still all excited about this "diet" of yours. You're literally fasting, and you've got it in your head that you need to do this every day or else you're failing at it altogether. You might have heard about some of the side effects, but don't really know if they affect everyone or not. Some people say it makes them tired, others say it makes them energetic. You may not feel much at all though since your body is just getting used to skipping a meal for the first time ever. You're still thinking about it though, and are trying to figure out the best way to do this.

What "break" is most appropriate? How many days should you fast? How much should you eat on the other days? And how do you feel when you start eating after fasting for a whole day or two (or more)? All these questions are arising in your head right now. You may be scared of these changes, but once they happen, they are a part of the process and make you stronger as well.

4. Acceptance

You've embraced this "diet" of yours, but there's still no set schedule on when to fast or how often. You do it when you feel like it and how you feel. Some days you'll fast a few hours and then eat well during the day. Others, you'll skip breakfast, lunch, and dinner altogether with only a snack here or there. There are no set rules or barriers as far as your diet goes at this point; it's just about finding what works for your body and eating according to that schedule. You begin to notice that some days are better than others. It's worth noting that all the negative effects of fasting are reversible physically when you resume eating regularly again, including bloating, headaches, fatigue, etc....

5. Stubbornness

You've already accepted the ups and downs of fasting as you go about your daily life, and realize that not every day is going to be great. You still enjoy this "diet," or whatever you want to call it. At this point, you're pretty much eating when you feel like it, but there's no longer a sense of fear or anxiety when you fast. You just go about your day normally without thinking about food or hunger at all because you know that if the body needs nutrition, hunger will kick in regardless of anything else going on in your life. And when it does kick in, any physical side effects are temporary and easily rectified with a meal.

6. Pessimism

You've been doing this "diet" of yours for a while now, and you're doing great! You forgot what it was like to eat six meals a day, but now you've got an "endless source of energy" thanks to those fast days. You're still fine with the lack of food on your schedule, and while you might miss a few occasional sweets every once in a while (which don't last long anyway), you feel great as far as dieting goes. One of the benefits is being able to sleep a lot better during those times when you don't have food for dinner anymore, but that's mostly out of habit from always eating so much before bedtime.

7. Non-Acceptance

You're at the point where you can't deal with fasting anymore. You thought it was going to be an easy diet, but now it's become a pain in the ass to do. But you've already accepted the fact that you feel great on fast days and eat normally on non-fasting days, but now you want more food during those days. You still get good sleep at night, but now you're tired during the day when you used to be energetic without eating breakfast or lunch. Your stomach has shrunken and every time your body feels hunger (which is often) you feel like you have a big hole in your stomach instead of an empty one. You don't know what to do anymore....

8. Pretty Much Nothing Is Different

You feel great, you sleep well, and you eat normally except during the two days a week when you're not eating. And then what? Same old diet with some "fasting" thrown in there? You feel like it's becoming a lot of work, and that's not really what you signed up for when you started the whole thing in the first place. You might want to continue it to get all the benefits of weight loss, but after a while it feels like nothing is different from where you were when you started.

9. The Solution

So... what's the solution? Shouldn't there be one? Well, yes and no. If you feel like fasting isn't changing anything, or if you feel like it's too much work, then by all means don't do it anymore. The best thing about fasting is that you're not depriving yourself of anything. If you're not losing weight, improving metabolism, sleeping better, and feeling better overall, then there isn't really a point to continue to do things the same way. But if you *can* keep doing this for the long run and all those wonderful benefits continue to come your way (or even get better), then why stop?

10. Conclusion

Fasting is a great way to shake things up and jump start your weight loss, but it's not something everyone can do. It's often easier for beginners than it is for those of us who have been doing it for years. Whatever you decide, I encourage you to make the decision based on your own experience, not on what someone else says (no matter how smart or wise they may seem).

CHAPTER 1: INTERMITTENT FASTING 101

> *"Everyone has a doctor in him; we just have to help him in his work. The natural healing force within each one of us is the greatest force in getting well. ...to eat when you are sick, is to feed your sickness."*
> *- Hippocrates*

What is in a name? That which we call intermittent fasting, the black sheep of the dieting world, by any other name would taste as sweet. Whether fasting for a day or for a week or more, this is one approach you might want to consider. What is intermittent fasting and why do some people get so riled up about it? It is an approach to dieting and eating that has been used for centuries and which is popular again today.

Let's start with the common ground: Intermittent fasting (IF) simply means that you go without food for a period of time. Maybe you take a break from eating between dinner one night and breakfast the next morning, or perhaps you fast for 24 hours on the weekend. Or maybe you do it every weekday for six months. Each approach has its own advantages and drawbacks (some of which we will get into later), but the important thing to understand is that it isn't just one way of dieting—it's many.

Here's the simplest way to think of it:

The more carbs you eat, the more insulin your body produces.

Insulin makes you fat—not directly, but indirectly. It tells your body to make more fat cells and holds on to fat cells that already exist. Insulin also tells you brain that it's time to make baby. No, not the reproductive kind of babies; I mean the making babies out of excess carbs and fat kind of babies. Your brain likes those because they are tasty and they help us get passed around and survive long enough to reproduce (in other words, we crave them). But eating a lot of them isn't exactly helping anyone move closer to their fitness goals.

On the other hand, low-carb eating triggers your body to release less insulin and makes you want to eat fewer carbs. The problem with this strategy—especially for people who are trying to lose weight—is that cutting out carbs also removes major nutrients like fiber, folate and many other vitamins and minerals from your diet.

Intermittent fasting is a viable alternative that is simple, safe and effective for losing weight (if you're doing it right) while keeping nutrient-rich whole foods in your diet.

Intermittent Fasting 101

The basic premise of intermittent fasting is that you take in all of your carbs and calories in a narrow window during the day (or on one day) and then fast through the other days. You also can do it every other day or every third day or pretty much any way you want. If you're trying to lose weight, it's best to do 16-hour fasts most days to keep your body from getting too used to eating during its fasting periods. It also helps prevent "starvation mode," a condition that causes your body to store more fat for future use when you go without food.

Here's how it works:

Let's say you choose to fast for 16 hours (for example, not eating anything after dinner one night and then having breakfast the next day at 10am). The other eight hours of the day, you "feed" yourself. In my case, I always do this by eating two meals that add up to about 1,600 calories. If you want to lose weight, aim for a total of 1,200 calories. Not only will your fasting days help your body to begin burning stored fats and reduce your insulin levels, but getting a few hundred extra calories each day also will help keep you from feeling too hungry and give you more energy to get through the fasts.

What you eat and when you eat it are important parts of the IF equation. You can eat whatever you want, but there are some simple guidelines to follow. First, the window of time between your last meal and your first one should be at least 16 hours. For example, don't eat anything after dinner one night and then start eating the next morning at 10am, 12 noon or 4pm. Whatever time you choose should be consistently adhered to on a daily basis. The second important factor is that your meals should include whole foods that aren't processed or refined. This isn't just about calories; it's about keeping your body healthy. Nutrient-rich foods help control insulin levels (which can prevent weight gain) and also help you stay satisfied between meals, which can make fasting easier over the long haul.

It's true that we digest our food more slowly as we get older and it helps to eat smaller meals throughout the day. That said, if you're starving yourself and going long periods of time between eating, your diet will not be as health-promoting or disease-preventing as it should be. You may also find that your energy levels are lower than they would be if you eat more frequently. Intermittent fasting is about keeping your body functioning at its best, day in and day out.

History of Intermittent Fasting

People have been fasting for as long as we have had recorded history. Fasts were once a common part of religious ceremonies and often included self-mortification (scourging, for example). Today most organized religions still observe special days of fasting, and a few require that all adherents follow certain dietary restrictions on those days. But for the most part, fasting has gone out of favor in modern society, replaced by diets like Atkins and other low-carb plans that allow people to eat frequently without going into ketosis.

As far back as 400 B.C., Hippocrates wrote about the therapeutic benefits of intermittent fasting—particularly when it was used with a low-carb diet to treat epilepsy and other diseases. And nearly every major ancient culture—from the Romans to the Greeks—recognized the health benefits of fasting.

Intermittent fasting also goes back many centuries in India. In Ayurveda, a system of traditional medicine, fasting is said to purify the body and rid it of toxins by restoring balance. The Ayurvedic fast is typically a period of 24 hours during which no food or water are consumed.

Fasting was first brought to the attention of modern Western science in the late 1800s. In one study conducted by a French physiologist named Germaine Cornaro, she fasted for 40 days (as observed by two physicians). She ate absolutely nothing during that time and afterwards was in robust health. When she resumed eating, her health quickly declined and she died at age 66.

Intermittent fasting has seen a rise in popularity recently—and for good reason. The research is more robust than ever, and it's clearer than ever that our bodies will function better without food than with it. Scientific studies are also proving that intermittent fasting can help to effectively treat health conditions and prevent disease, such as diabetes, obesity, heart disease and many cancers.

The modern lifestyle offers so many tasty food options. But a diet that is filled with processed foods, fast foods, baked goods and other sweets is a diet that tends to lead to obesity, diabetes and heart disease. Instead of trying to eat fewer calories, intermittent fasting encourages people to eat less often—and research indicates that it can help you live longer and enjoy better health as well. We're living in an age where fast food and processed foods are the norm. The modern lifestyle makes it difficult to live a healthy life.

Intermittent fasting vs Calorie restriction diets

Intermittent fasting is quite different from other diets because it's typically a shorter period of time.

When people make changes to their diet, they often feel motivated for a few weeks. But then the motivation tends to fade as they get busy with work or family obligations or lose focus on what they're trying to accomplish. Intermittent fasting can help you push past those moments when you lose focus and get back on track. There are several studies comparing intermittent fasting to calorie restriction, which is considered the gold standard for weight loss. And while intermittent fasting can be a great tool in your weight loss arsenal—especially if used combined with exercise and healthy eating—it's not an alternative to proper nutrition.

Calorie restriction diets work because they're focused on creating a deficit of 3,500 calories over the course of three to four weeks. This results in weight loss of about 1 pound for every week that you restrict your calories. Intermittent fasting is designed to create a deficit through calorie restriction, but over a period of just 24 hours or less. While this can help you lose weight quickly, it's also not an easy task to accomplish. It requires careful meal planning and preparation to ensure that you're getting the right amount of nutrients each day. Most importantly, Calorie restriction isn't a long-term diet plan because it doesn't teach you how to maintain your new weight or lifestyle permanently.

IF on the other hand is sustainable — most studies have shown that people who practice it regularly are able maintain their weight loss and healthy lifestyle for many years. It's also a great diet for people to stay on after they've reached their goals because you can eat anything you want as long as you track it — no more calorie counting or worrying about portion control.

One of the biggest differences between intermittent fasting and other popular diets is that with intermittent fasting, you eat whatever you want. Yes, you read that correctly. You can eat as many calories as you like in a single day with intermittent fasting, and there are no meal plans or strict guidelines to follow.

Seasoned IF veterans may scoff at this and insist that you will not get the same results if you eat fast food or pizza. But it's important to remember that they've been fasting regularly for a long time, so their bodies are adapted to functioning on fewer calories. If you're just starting out, then slowly "re-introduce" different foods into your diet to see how your body responds and if certain foods cause any negative side effects.

Finally, and most importantly, IF is enjoyable.

CHAPTER 2: INTERMITTENT FASTING AND AGING

Physical changes don't stop when you reach fifty years old. While they might not be as dramatic, there are noticeable differences in how your body will look and react to certain things as you get older. Weight gain is one of these changes, with fat collecting around the stomach and hips. Muscle loss is another inevitable consequence of getting older which can be caused by a lack of activity or "use it or lose it." The skin also begins to thin as cells die off, resulting in wrinkles, dryness, age spots and liver spots.

The good thing is that we are living longer than ever before. People in the 21st century are living longer, healthier lives than any previous generation in history. There are many who even reach the 100-year-old mark. Our bodies have adapted to change over long periods of time. The way we live now is different (no pun intended) from the way people lived hundreds of years ago. Part of aging gracefully is accepting that your body is not going to look or act like it used to when you were a teenager or young adult, but this doesn't mean you're going to be less healthy or less capable of living life as fully as you can.

<u>The hair</u>

The hair is not immune to age-related changes either. The hair has the same color pigmentation as the skin, only it's much more concentrated and visible. The hair will begin to lose its pigment and become increasingly more transparent until it disappears altogether. As women age, there is a corresponding loss of vascularity in the scalp, making their hair grow slower or thinner than before.

The thyroid gland slows down at this point as well, which can cause thinning or baldness in some people. The thyroid regulates your body's metabolism and controls the production of your hormones. If the gland isn't producing enough hormones, your metabolism will slow down and you'll gain weight. Thyroid problems are one of the most common complaints associated with aging.

The skin

Your skin will begin to lose elasticity as you get older, causing it to sag and wrinkle. You will probably notice wrinkles around your eyes, mouth and neck first, mainly because they are areas that show expression. Your skin will also begin to dry out as it loses the natural oils within it. This change can be slowed by drinking plenty of water and using a moisturizer twice a day.

The veins in our body become less visible as we age just like our hair, becoming more transparent until they eventually disappear. The muscle tissue itself begins to shrink and atrophy from lack of use or overuse injuries like sprains and strains. If you used to be very active but have begun to sit in the chair more often, the muscles will become weaker and will shrink in size.

Tendons and ligaments are also affected by sports injuries or aging and can begin to tear more easily than when you were younger. This can result in joint pain and difficulty moving around. Your bones age too, just like your teeth do. You can live healthy all your life, but once you reach an advanced age, there is nothing that can stop osteoporosis from taking its toll on your skeletal system. Bones become more porous as they lose minerals and calcium, which makes them weaker and easier to break.

The heart

The heart isn't immune to age-related changes either. The membrane around the heart, called the pericardium, tends to become inflamed with age. This is called pericarditis and can be caused by an infection or by disease. The heart muscle itself will begin to lose its ability to contract and relax as a result of years of working and pumping blood throughout your body. The muscle tissue itself becomes less elastic and less resilient over time, which makes it more difficult for the heart to pump blood efficiently. When a person is in their forties or fifties and begins to experience angina, it could mean there is an underlying problem with their heart.

Your heart will also begin to pump less blood per beat as you get older. This can lead to symptoms like fatigue, dizziness and chest pain, but if left unchecked can also lead to a more serious illness such as heart failure or stroke.

The digestive system

The way your body digests food will change as well. Your metabolism slows down dramatically in your later years, so you can't eat as much as before without gaining weight. You will probably need to cut back on the amount of fat and sugar you take in daily too. If you notice a change in the consistency of your stool, this could mean you have developed an infection or are suffering from constipation.

Hormones and internal organs

There are many other changes that take place as you get older. You will notice the onset of menopause in your late 40s or early 50s, marked by hot flashes, night sweats, insomnia and mood swings. The adrenal glands produce less hormones as we age which can lead to fatigue and weight gain. The ovaries stop producing eggs and begin to shrink, and the pituitary gland stops releasing sex hormones like estrogen and progesterone which can lead to sexual disorders such as low libido or vaginal dryness.

The internal organs themselves will begin to shrink and atrophy as they are not used as often. The kidneys can take a lot of damage from things like high blood pressure or diabetes, which can lead to kidney disease. The heart muscles can weaken and the kidneys will shrink as well, making it more difficult for them to filter out toxins and excess fluids. The liver produces less bile, making it harder for the body to break down fats and digest food. This can lead to various digestion problems including constipation and gas.

You can try to slow down these changes by making healthy choices and staying active as you get older. You'll want to take it easy and not overdo things, especially as your heart ages. It may be best to go for a walk around the block instead of a jog, or limit your time at the gym. Remember that you can't stay young and active forever. You can slow down these changes by making healthy choices and staying active as you get older. You'll want to take it easy and not overdo things, especially as your heart ages. It may be best to go for a walk around the block instead of a jog, or limit your time at the gym.

Slowing down these changes with intermittent fasting

There are a number of ways to help the body cope with its changes and one of these methods is intermittent fasting. Intermittent fasting is a simple way to alter your eating habits in order to give your body some relief as you get older. It is also one of the healthiest ways to lose weight or keep it off, especially when you are focusing on healthy foods and cutting out processed junk. Fasting and caloric restriction is the most effective way to optimize your longevity. Few people understand how fasting, which only means going without food for a particular time period, can be beneficial to the hair, skin, and nails. Reducing the number of calories, you eat each day can lead to longer lasting hair, nails, and skin.

This is because when you eat these extra calories, your body turns the extra food into fat and stores it under the skin, around the eyes, and on other parts of the body. This can lead to more wrinkles, larger breasts, puffier cheeks and eye circles, skin tags, sagging arms and legs, cellulite, spider veins in your face or legs, and other unsightly body changes.

When you reduce your caloric intake by fasting for some time each day for a few days each week, you will burn off those excess calories that your body was storing away. You will also be eating less food which means you won't have to worry about constipation or feeling bloated after a meal.

CHAPTER 3: WHAT INTERMITTENT FASTING DOES

The concept of intermittent fasting is nothing new. The idea—eating only during an 8-hour window a day, for example—was first popularized in 2005 with the bestseller, Eat Stop Eat. Intermittent fasting has now been shown to have many benefits, from weight loss to improved cognition and longevity.

Intermittent fasting is not a diet in the typical sense; it's more of a pattern of eating that may be good for your brain as well as your waistline. It can also help keep you healthy when combined with other healthy lifestyle habits such as regular exercise and plenty of sleep.

Intermittent fasting is a pattern of eating that fits in naturally with your body's circadian rhythms. Our ancestors went to bed when it got dark and rose with the sun. This helped them use energy from food more efficiently, to better sustain their bodies and brains. In turn, this helped them live longer and be healthier overall. We live in a very different world today—with 24/7 access to food and distractions like Facebook—so our eating patterns are out of sync with our body clocks. That can lead to weight gain.

Intermittent fasting can help give you more energy, more clarity, better sleep, and more balanced blood-sugar levels. Why? It's all about managing your insulin levels by controlling when you eat. If you don't eat for a period of time—while also avoiding high-carbohydrate foods—your blood sugar will stabilize and your insulin will drop. This can lead to better fat burning and overall health.

ACCELERATES WEIGHT LOSS

Fasting is not a diet, but rather a pattern of eating that is good for your brain as well as your waistline. It can help keep you healthy when combined with other healthy lifestyle habits such as regular exercise and plenty of sleep. Intermittent fasting can help you lose weight because it reduces the amount of insulin your body produces, which helps your body burn fat instead of storing it. Studies have shown that intermittent fasting can be an effective way to lose weight. One of the most-cited studies was published in 2004, which looked at the effect of alternate-day fasting on adults who were overweight or obese. The goal was to determine whether this pattern of eating could improve weight loss and maintenance when added to a calorie-restricted diet. Over the course of each 3-month intervention, participants lost an average of 8 percent of their body weight (about 35 pounds per person) and maintained most of their lean muscle mass.

Another study, published in 2012, looked at the effects of alternate-day fasting on weight loss in a group of obese adults who were put on a diet and exercise regularly. Each participant was given a personal goal of losing at least 10 pounds each month. The group that followed the alternate-day fasting diet lost an average of more than 14 pounds—more than double what the control group without fasting lost over the same period.

When you eat food, you store some of the calories as fat. The more food you eat, the more fat you store. When you fast—that is, when you don't eat for 20 hours or so—you allow your body to use fat as an energy source instead of storing it. You can also control when your body uses stored fat as a fuel. This is important because it gives your body the chance to burn off excess fat that is not needed for immediate energy requirements. By giving your body regular access to stored body fat, which would otherwise be inaccessible due to continuous eating, intermittent fasting ensures that your body can burn off excess fat.

IMPROVES COGNITIVE FUNCTION

Some critics argue that fasting can have adverse effects on your brain, especially if you do it too frequently. But several studies have shown that intermittent fasting is not detrimental to brain health. In an April 2013 study, researchers found that alternate-day fasting had a beneficial effect on human participants' learning and memory. The study also found that fasting increased the overall number of new nerve connections in the hippocampus, which is where short-term memory is stored and long-term memories are formed. These new nerve connections might be linked with improved thinking ability and better performance on cognitive tests. This suggests that intermittent fasting can help improve memory loss and enhance cognitive function.

Another study, published in January 2015 in the journal Frontiers in Aging Neuroscience, found that alternate-day fasting may even protect the brains of elderly people who are at risk for Alzheimer's disease. The researchers followed 20 healthy adults aged 65 to 85 for eight weeks, putting half of them on a modified version of alternate-day fasting and half on a regular diet with no restrictions. The results showed significant improvements in verbal memory with no adverse effects from the dietary intervention. The researchers suggest that alternate-day fasting might be beneficial to elderly people who need to ward off the early signs of dementia and brain degeneration associated with Alzheimer's disease.

HELPS MANAGE DIABETES

Intermittent fasting also has therapeutic potential in the treatment and management of diabetes. Fasting is especially helpful for type 2 diabetics. It helps regulate blood sugar, allowing your body to use insulin more efficiently, which reduces the amount of insulin needed to keep your blood sugar levels in check. Intermittent fasting is not recommended for those who are prediabetic or insulin resistant—in this case, eating small meals every few hours will still help control blood sugar levels and reduce insulin resistance.

One study published in the journal Nutrition & Metabolism showed that intermittent fasting was more effective at reducing body weight than regular calorie restriction. For the study, researchers split 10 overweight adults with type 2 diabetes into two groups. The first group followed a 20-hour-per-day fasting schedule for three months. The second group followed a typical 24-hour eating schedule for three months. At the end of the experiment, both groups had lost an average of 10 pounds, but the intermittent fasting group lost significantly more—about 14 pounds versus just six for the regular calorie restriction participants.

BOOSTS KETONE PRODUCTION

Ketosis is a natural metabolic process in which your body burns fat instead of glucose for fuel. In this state, called ketosis, your body produces ketones—small fatty acids that provide your body with energy. Intermittent fasting induces ketosis, allowing you to get the benefits of this normally very unpleasant metabolic process without suffering through the negative side effects like nausea and fatigue.

Your body normally uses glucose as its primary source of fuel, but when you're eating a ketogenic diet, which is extremely low in net carbs (less than 20 grams per day), your body begins to burn fat instead. Once in the state of ketosis, your body actually can't produce and use glucose anymore, so you become completely dependent on fat for energy. And when you have no carbohydrates left in your body, you produce ketones instead. The best part is that when you become fat-adapted, keto-adapted, or "keto"— the state of running on ketones—your brain loves it. This means there's no discomfort or slowdown in cognitive function. You can run on ketones indefinitely.

BALANCES HORMONES

Research shows that intermittent fasting can help regulate hormone levels, reducing the risk of diabetes and other metabolic diseases in women. What's more, intermittent fasting helps reduce insulin resistance and inflammation over time (two of the main causes of type 2 diabetes).

The research shows that when you regularly fast, your body adapts to the fasting state. This means that you can probably increase the frequency of your fasts or decrease them over time.

INCREASES YOUR WILLPOWER

Intermittent fasting is actually quite easy once you get past the initial adjustment stage, because you're doing it only as long as it takes for your body to switch over into using fat for fuel. And once you're in the feeding phase, hunger becomes easier to manage. You'll still get a good amount of calories in, and even more importantly, you'll be satiated for much longer periods of time than before—because fat lasts a lot longer as your body's fuel source than glucose does. Once daily intermittent fasting means that many people who have previously struggled with diets can hold out for hours and hours before feeling the need to feed again.

And as far as hunger goes, it's important to note that even though intermittent fasting is more a means of extending the length of time you go without eating than it is about restricting calories, your body doesn't know the difference. This means you can enjoy big feasts—so long as you have the discipline to fit them into a short window of time.

IT'S A NATURAL THERAPY FOR GERD

Because it can be hard to tell if what you're experiencing is a symptom of something more serious, it's important to take any concerns about changes in your health seriously. That said, heartburn (gastroesophageal reflux disease or GERD) is one of the most common ailments faced by people who are over 50 years old—and more than half of people with GERD also suffer from frequent indigestion. While occasional heartburn may not be too concerning, frequent heartburn could be a sign that you're not getting enough fiber in your diet–and eating fiber-rich foods helps reduce the symptoms of GERD.

PREVENTS OSTEOPOROSIS

There is evidence that intermittent fasting can reduce your risk of certain cancers, including the most common types of breast cancer (invasive ductal carcinoma and invasive lobular carcinoma). Not only do the changes in how a person's body handles insulin thanks to intermittent fasting help prevent cancer cells from growing, but research in both humans and animals shows that intermittent fasting also reduces levels of insulin-like growth factor 1 (IGF-1) in the blood. And higher levels of IGF-1 have been linked with a greater risk of multiple types of cancer.

HELPS YOU LIVE LONGER

Intermittent fasting has been shown to protect against the harmful effects of aging in both the body and brain. One study found that intermittent fasting decreased oxidative damage to protein structures in the brain, which prevents cells from getting damaged and fosters healthier brain function over time. Other studies have found that intermittent fasting protects animals from developing age-related cognitive impairment, and can help control Alzheimer's disease and Parkinson's disease.

In one study published in 2016, researchers found that intermittent fasting helped reduce the risk factors associated with metabolic syndrome. The study revealed that intermittent fasting lowered triglyceride levels and improved cholesterol levels. Since high blood pressure is usually paired with high cholesterol, this is good news for people who struggle to control their blood pressure.

Intermittent fasting has been shown to reduce oxidative stress and inflammation, which plays a role in many aging-related diseases. When you eat food, your body breaks down what you eat into glucose or carbohydrates (glycogen) for energy. The glycogen is then stored in your liver and muscles to be used when your body needs energy. When glycogen stores are full, the extra glucose is turned into fat, and that's stored in the body as well.

BETTER CARDIOVASCULAR FUNCTION

Intermittent fasting also has a beneficial effect on blood pressure, cholesterol and triglycerides—all risk factors for heart disease. And since healthy arteries help lower blood pressure, intermittent fasting may help both to keep blood pressure within normal bounds and reduce the risk of heart attack and stroke. A study published in the journal Circulation showed that intermittent fasting lowered blood pressure in people with type 2 diabetes more than a conventional was similar to daily calorie restriction, although intermittent fasting did result in greater reductions in insulin resistance.

<u>What intermittent doesn't do</u>

Intermittent fasting (IF) is far from a new concept. In fact, it has been around for centuries and known to many ancient cultures including the Egyptians, the Native Americans, and the Greeks. The benefits of intermittent fasting are now being realized by people all over the world who are realizing that they can eat whatever they choose but cut their calorie intake intermittently in order to reach their weight loss goals.

However just because intermittent fasting isn't new doesn't mean there aren't myths about it that have managed to permeate into society at large. Here are some of the most common myths about intermittent fasting that you need to be aware of before you begin your own IF journey.

INTERMITTENT FASTING WILL SLOW YOUR METABOLISM

This is probably the most common myth about intermittent fasting and it's one that many people struggle with when they first decide to give IF a try. While it is true that IF will slow down your metabolism (remember, we're not talking about eating nothing here, just eating less) it will actually speed it back up once you return to normal eating patterns. It seems counterintuitive but this is how many different diets work. The body regulates metabolism based on caloric intake and IF causes a slight calorie restriction so the body slows down metabolism but once you return to normal eating patterns then you can speed things up a little again.

IF BURNS MUSCLES, NOT FAT

One of the biggest misconceptions about intermittent fasting is that it causes your body to go into starvation mode. In this mode, your muscle mass decreases as your body goes all out trying to burn fat. However, research shows that very low-calorie diets can help you burn fat and not muscle. One study found that two groups of dieters— one group following a traditional diet, the other following an alternate-day fasting diet—decreased their abdominal fat and increased their lean muscle mass over a period of six months.

IF WILL MESS WITH YOUR SLEEPING PATTERNS

While it is true that you may have an initial period of disorientation when transitioning to an IF lifestyle, overall, you should see improvements in your sleeping patterns. A study that was done at the University of Chicago found that skipping breakfast did not negatively impact the quality and duration of sleep-in individuals who followed a fasting plan over a two-week span. If anything, participants felt less tired and more alert during the day while they ate only one meal per day. Adhering to this plan will help you improve your sleeping patterns along with improving other aspects of your health as well.

IF MAKES YOU WEAK

While it is true that IF can make your stomach grumble and growl when you are in a fasting state, it does not mean that you will have low energy. Actually, the opposite is usually true. Because your body knows that it doesn't have as many calories to work with, it tends to store what few calories there are away in the muscles and this can increase your overall energy levels. You may initially find yourself feeling tired after eating a small meal but once your body starts burning off those stored calories than your energy levels will increase.

CHAPTER 3: TYPES OF INTERMITTENT FASTING

"He who eats until he is sick must fast until he is well

-Anonymous

One Meal a Day

Many people know it as OMAD fasting, others prefer to call it a one meal a day diet. Whatever you call it, this is not a new concept. It is the idea that you can lose weight by eating just one meal per day and eschewing any other snacks or food. While it may sound counterintuitive to eat only once a day, many people have tried it and found that it does work. Before you consider OMAD, however, there are things you should know.

WHAT IS ONE MEAL A DAY?

One meal a day is the fast track to weight loss and many studies have confirmed that. It also happens to be a good way to live a healthy lifestyle. It helps you keep your calories down while at the same time losing weight faster than if you were eating three meals per day. This type of dieting should only be done until you reach your goal weight, but for some people, this can last for life.

To be able to do this type of dieting, you need to eat a lot of protein. This will keep your body from feeling hungry as quickly. However, you also need to make sure that you are eating the right kinds of protein. Lean meats and fish are best for this kind of eating plan. They should be cooked lightly and in a healthy manner, without adding fats or oils that would slow down weight loss.

You should also consider the amount of calories that you burn during the day. You obviously burn calories when you exercise, but there are other activities that will burn calories as well. For instance, walking around town can burn about 100 calories per hour if you do it regularly. Having an active lifestyle will also help you to lose weight. This is why many people that use OMAD find that it works really well.

Your daily allowance should be somewhere between 1,000 and 1,500 calories a day. This should help you lose weight quickly without taking the joy out of eating. In addition to this, keep in mind that if you do not eat enough calories, your body will go into the same type of hibernation that it does during sleep. As such, you need to make sure that you are eating enough carbohydrates and proteins so it does not go into this mode. A good way to get the right amount of calories is to eat three meals a day, but cut your portions in half. If you do not like the idea of cutting your portions in half, you should try eating just one meal at night.

THE BENEFITS OF ONE MEAL A DAY

Some people will tell you that eating only once a day will keep you from becoming hungry. However, that is not really true for most people. Once your body gets used to this type of dieting, it will feel hungry less often and faster when it does feel hunger. You simply have to give your body time to adjust and then it will work just fine as long as you are taking in enough protein.

Another benefit to eating this way is that it is much easier to stop eating once you are full. Many people find that after they have eaten fewer calories for a while, they stop feeling hungry in the middle of a meal. This makes it easy to eat less and lose weight. It also keeps you from getting too full when you are eating an actual meal with family or friends.

You will also be more aware of what your body is telling you because your stomach will tell you when it is time to eat again. This is a much better way to lose weight than trying to get your body used to smaller portions.

OMAD is ideal for women over 50 who need to lose weight quickly before hitting that big birthday. If you are trying to lose 50 pounds in a year, one meal a day is the fastest way to do it without starving yourself or doing an extreme diet. Just remember that it is not a permanent way of eating. Once you have reached your goal weight, shift back to a normal eating schedule with three meals per day. This will ensure that you stay healthy and keep the weight off long-term.

Sure, OMAD fasting may be an odd way of eating, but when it comes down to it, it is not a bad way. Eat a lot of protein, keep your calories down, and you will see yourself losing weight quickly. It is also a nice change of pace from the daily grind.

Alternate Day Fasting

Like many radical diets, we've already been doing it for years. Slight modifications in the frequency of our meals or the length of time we spend in fasted state can make us leaner and healthier.

It's called Alternate day fasting (ADF) and the concept is quite simple: you consume nothing but water (or low-calorie drinks) every other day, while on 'feeding days' you can eat to your heart's content. The so called 'feeding days' are supposed to be performed weekly, although many people combine this with a 5:2 diet (5 days of ADF alternating with 2 'normal' eating days) which we will be looking at next.

The idea is that our bodies needs at least 12 hours to digest food properly. This is a basic biological fact that even a caveman knew. You can't just gorge yourself all day long, then go to sleep and expect your body to cleanse and repair itself within the next 8 hours - it will simply not happen, no matter how good your digestion is.

Therefore, the premise of ADF is simple: you eat today and fast tomorrow. A typical ADF schedule would have an individual fast for 24 hours, followed by one 'feed day' (24 hours of eating) and another 24 hours fast. The frequency can be increased to three-day-long fasts once the individual has lost a certain amount of weight/body fat - again, depending on the specific fitness goals.

This schedule can be adjusted slightly, with the fast being reduced to 18 hours, for example.

Pros of Alternate Day Fast:

• A natural way to lose weight. The idea is that by alternating between feast and famine you will be able to lose weight while your body is in a calorie deficit state. • Less hunger than traditional diets - hunger is known to be one of the main reasons why people quit their diet plans. With ADF you'll end up experiencing less hunger pangs than on a regular diet, which makes it easier for you to stay on track. • Based on scientific research - I know, strange as it sounds.

This is a good thing for several reasons

As we've established already, your body needs at least 12 hours to process food and get ready for the next meal. So, if you eat breakfast at 8:00 am today, you'll be hungry before bedtime and will need to eat a substantial snack in order to sleep until morning. That's not ideal.

Intermittent fasting (which is what ADF is) has been scientifically proven to raise human growth hormone levels. This is a key element in building lean muscle mass, decreasing body fat levels and improving overall health.

When following ADF your insulin levels will be much more stable (insulin spikes are one of the main reasons for weight gain/obesity). It also makes it easier to lose weight, because when you're eating less regularly insulin sensitivity increases as well.

However, this isn't a 'magic' solution - it's just another tool you can use in your arsenal against obesity and related health problems.

A word of caution: If you're going to try ADF, don't expect it to be a walk in the park. Since your body goes into short periods of famine when following this diet, it's bound to cause some hunger and cravings. It might also give you headaches, mood swings and other side effects - but these are temporary!

ADF is best for women, post-menopausal women, the elderly and anyone with medical issues. If you're young and physically active, you probably won't benefit from following ADF.

The 5:2 diet

This one is a bit more complicated than the two diets above. The idea behind this one is to eat 'normally' five days a week and then to restrict your calorie intake to just 500-600 calories during the other two days of the week.

You can choose what to eat and when. It's up to you whether you want to fast 2 days a week or 5 days a week. You don't have to eat the same thing on both fasting days.

The time span of the fasts and the overall caloric intake differ slightly between people who follow this diet.

Fasting is not a diet for beginners. It is recommended that you try shorter fasts of 12 to 16 hours before embarking on the four-day fast. If you don't have any experience with fasting, at least do an overnight fast once a week, like sleeping overnight without eating anything.

If you've never done a seven-day water fast – don't start with this. You can however complete several shorter fasts of 3-5 days each before attempting a long one. You will need to prepare for it and get used to it.

Eat-Stop-Eat Intermittent Fasting

This type of intermittent fasting is very similar to the 16/8 method that we've talked about earlier.

In this case however, you are not eating for one continuous period of time, but rather for 24 hours and then not eating for the next 24 hours. So, there are two 12 hour fasting periods every day.

The Eat-Stop-Eat diet is recommended if you want to follow a very low-calorie diet (VLCD) in order to lose weight quickly, but still want to make sure that you don't lose muscle mass.

Because the Eat-Stop-Eat fasts are quite short, there's no problem with muscle loss and you can even lift weights when doing ESE if you wish.

In order to complete an ESE fast you have to use a 24-hour clock. You can start your fast at any time of the day, but once you stop eating you must wait until the next 12-hour period has started before resuming with food.

Which one to choose – OMAD, ADF or ESE?

The answer to this question is not a simple one. All three different types of intermittent fasting have their pros and cons, which we will explore in this article. However, we do believe that periodic use of the OMAD or ADF protocol could be better for women over 50 years old. As always, consult with your doctor before starting an intermittent fasting program to make sure it is safe for you.

OMAD: In the OMAD protocol, you eat all your daily food within an 8-hour time window during your day (such as 12pm-8pm). This type of intermittent fasting was shown to improve insulin sensitivity and blood sugar levels in people with type 2 diabetes who were eating too many carbs. With the OMAD protocol, fasting blood sugar levels were even lower. However, this means that you may have blood sugar swings and go hypoglycemic during or between meals. You may also have some nutrient deficiencies, so it is not recommended for women over 50 years old. Another downside of OMAD is that you will be eating different foods every day. This can cause boredom and hunger cravings.

ADF: In the ADF protocol (All Day Fasting), you can eat all your daily food (vegan-meal plan) at the same time – although this usually results in losing weight quickly because of higher calorie consumption. Some women experience hormone and metabolic shifts while fasting. It has been shown that women over 50 years old may have more problems with weight loss while on an ADF protocol. This is because the way our bodies work slows down after certain age and we are less metabolically efficient in burning fuel (fat). Although, a study found that the women who fasted for 24 hours had lower fasting glucose levels than those in the control group. The reason why we think intermittent fasting is better for older women is because it helps you break the pattern of regulating your hunger by eating every 2-3 hours and you will have better energy levels during your fast. Older women should note, however, that if you are elderly and your health is not the best, using ADF may result in the opposite – poor health and low energy levels.

ESE: In this eating schedule a person eats 25-30% of their daily calories one time during the day (such as 8am-5pm). You can eat whatever you wish within this 8-hour window. This is the best choice for women over 50 years old. It can help with weight loss and improve energy levels. Also, it reduces food cravings, hunger, and brain fog (those pesky feelings of "brain fog" that often happen in the early morning hours after eating a big meal at night).

So, which one to choose? This depends on your goals as well as how healthy you are. If you are healthy and your goals include weight loss, then ESE is definitely the best choice for women over 50 years. If your goal is to be healthy and avoid gaining weight, OMAD may be a better fit.

CHAPTER 4: GETTING STARTED WITH INTERMITTENT FASTING

Fasting isn't just for young people with hours of metabolism in their favor. Women over 50 can use fasting as well: just gradually ease into it to avoid risks.

If you're a woman over the age of 50 and have been thinking about intermittent fasting, you might be concerned about health precautions. The truth is, studies have shown that fasting can actually promote longevity and prevent disease. When done properly, it can even help you lose weight, contributing to a longer, healthier life.

Although there are some health precautions that you should take into consideration when fasting, they are best addressed by having a doctor or nutritionist review your health history and answer any questions you might have about the process.

It's important to remember that over the years your body has likely gone through many changes and no two bodies will react exactly the same to fasting. This chapter presents some of the most common concerns women over 50 have about using intermittent fasting as a part of their weight loss routine but also includes tips on how to overcome them in order to achieve greater and faster lasting results.

The list of problems and medical conditions associated with fasting is extensive. Some of the most common symptoms include low blood pressure, loss of appetite, dizziness, light-headedness and feeling faint. Although these problems are easily avoidable when fasting properly, it's still important to work closely with a doctor or dietician to ensure that you don't have any underlying issues that might prevent you from safely fasting.

Fasting can be dangerous for pregnant women and women who are nursing their children; they should in no way participate in this type of diet. Women who are obese and older than 50 may be at risk for osteoporosis during a fast as well as those who have some form of heart disease or diabetes.

The following are just a few of the most common health concerns that women over 50 have about fasting and how to overcome those concerns.

#1: Will I lose muscle mass faster than fat?

Most women worry that their bodies use up muscle mass as they age. Unfortunately, after menopause, muscle mass decreases by about one pound every year. This is especially true of the muscles in your arms and legs because it's harder to maintain muscle in those areas than it is in the middle of your body.

When you have adequate nutrition and a healthy lifestyle, you may be able to hold off aging symptoms for several years longer than your peers. But as you age, losing muscle mass is inevitable. This doesn't mean that fat loss will be the same for everyone though; those with fast metabolism and a high level of insulin sensitivity won't be able to lose any muscle mass no matter what they do.

#2: Can I eat too much fat?

It may help to understand the difference between eating to lose weight and eating for weight maintenance or weight gain. Eating for maintenance or weight gain will cause your body to store fat more efficiently than those who are eating in order to decrease body weight.

If you want to maintain a healthy weight, it's best not to focus on how many calories you're using up each day but rather think about the quality of your food. Eating a lot of protein, healthy fats and good carbohydrates will slow down the absorption of calories and help you feel full longer.

Intermittent fasting is often recommended for those struggling with overeating or obesity. While it may actually help maintain a healthier body weight, most women over 50 are eating for weight loss anyway. If you're eating more than 2,000 calories per day with the intention of losing fat, you may be in danger of increasing your caloric intake to much higher levels than a woman over 50 should be at.

Planning for intermittent fasting

If you're not already familiar with fasting, it's important to consult with a physician or nutritionist before attempting any type of fast. A proper plan can make a big difference in helping you successfully complete your first fast.

Fast for 16 hours then eat for 8 hours with a daily caloric intake of 1,200 to 1,300 calories.

The following fasting tips should help you have an easier time starting intermittent fasting while keeping your body intact and injury free:

BE PREPARED

Time your meals so that when the fast starts and when it ends, all you need to do is grab something easy from the refrigerator or pantry. If you allow yourself to get too hungry, it can be very difficult to concentrate on your work or get anything done.

Before your first fast, you can try practicing intermittent fasting for a few days by skipping one meal or eating only twice a day. For example, skip your morning coffee and breakfast but make sure to eat lunch and then dinner before the fast begins.

This way you'll be able to get an idea of how much energy you have throughout the day without eating and learn how long it takes for your brain to feel hungry again. If you're not used to skipping meals often or in this manner, it's best not to begin fasting until you've had some experience with how eating less frequently affects your body and mind.

Most of the time you'll need to begin fasting on an empty stomach to feel hungry again quickly; however, don't try this if your last meal contained alcohol or spicy foods. In addition, make sure that your dinner isn't loaded with carbohydrates and fat so that you aren't too full while you sleep.

CONSIDER A NO-FASTING DAY OR TWO

Even if you're able to fast without any negative side effects, it's still a good idea to use your first few fasts as an opportunity to experiment with eating at least two days a week.

It's fine if you don't follow through with every fast, especially if you're just starting out. You may feel that it's best for your health to spend a few weeks or months eating more often but eventually you'll be able to determine your personal fasting schedule.

OBTAIN PROPER NUTRITION AND REST

If you're attempting a 24-hour water fast, make sure that the last meal of your day is eaten well before bedtime. Eat something nutritious (not overly full of fat and carbohydrates) and drink a large amount of water during the hour leading up to bedtime so that when hunger begins to set in, there are enough nutrients in your body to keep you going for at least three or four hours.

If you're attempting a multi-day fast or one in which you'll be fasting while walking or working outside, make sure to eat plenty of fruits when they're in season and take the time to schedule breaks for food and rest. If you feel light-headed or weak from hunger, take the time to sit down and eat something so that you aren't forced to stop the fast for a meal. Fasting should never be exhausting or uncomfortable, so make certain that you're getting enough of what your body needs during the day so that it's easy to continue.

Making massive changes in your diet or attempting things like fasting too soon before going on vacation can be very stressful and detrimental to your overall health, so don't rush it. Focus on eating healthier foods over time instead of drastically changing your routine right away.

When you're eating every other day, don't be afraid of trying new foods or preparing meals in different ways. You deserve a break from the same old foods that you've been eating for years. Don't be afraid to approach your food planning differently than you normally would, and don't forget to enjoy it!

ADD SOME EXERCISE

If possible, try to do some form of exercise before beginning your first fast so that your body is prepared for what lies ahead. Whether you work out during the week or not, you're going to be burning far more calories than normal while fasting and it would be a good idea to prepare your body in some way.

Just a few minutes each day are enough to begin with and as you get used to doing so, you can increase the length of your workouts until you feel at optimal health. This way, when you do fast, your body doesn't experience any loss of energy and is able to keep up its normal functions.

Walking is an excellent form of exercise for weight loss that doesn't require any special equipment or training. You can also try doing some aerobic exercises during the weekend if you're accustomed to working out at this time.

When it comes to the weight loss benefits of fasting, there's no shortage of information and studies have proven that a prolonged period of fasting can lead to a significant weight loss.

The only thing you'll need is a dehydrator and some food – yes, you can still go through the process of fasting even if you're at work! You just need to make sure you always have snacks with you so that your body won't get too hungry all the time. You will also need to know when you should drink water, as well as what kinds of foods you should and shouldn't consume.

Always remember to eat breakfast, snack on protein-rich foods throughout the day, get a good night's sleep and drink a lot of water. This isn't too hard and will help you not only look skinny but also be healthy. There are many ways for you to lose weight rapidly, but the best method is through dieting and exercising properly.

<u>Boosting energy levels with intermittent fasting</u>

At 50. many people experience more sluggishness. In a world where people are working 10 hours a day or more, the 8-hour work day is not always the norm. Added to this, when we age our bodies produce less human growth hormone (HGH), which is thought to contribute to slow metabolic rates and weight gain.

Are you having too much or too little?

To figure out how much to limit food intake, try using calorie tracking software or consulting with a nutritionist — even a health professional who is trained in intermittent fasting can help. However, if you are uncomfortable tracking food intake or estimating your caloric needs, then another way to determine when to eat is by answering these questions:

1. Do I feel like I am starving? If so, this indicates that you are not eating enough calories and your body is running out of fuel.

2. Do I feel like I am not hungry at all? If so, this indicates that you are eating too much and your body is storing food as fat.

3. How do I feel? If you feel good, energized and not hungry at all, chances are you don't need to eat any more. Otherwise, take a small break and then eat again when you feel the urge to do so. The best way to sustain this form of dieting is by setting up a routine for yourself – try scheduling times for meals because it makes it easier to remember when it is time to eat/drink. When it comes to intermittent fasting, learn how to eliminate the "food coma" that can happen when you skip meals and monitor what you feel like eating.

HIGH CALORIE INTERMITTENT FASTING

I recommend using the ketogenic diet plan. It is a low carbohydrate, high fat, high protein plan and can help you with weight loss. For those who are interested in intermittent fasting, try to go half-way between your eating window. For example, if you normally fast for 12 hours and eat all day or eat 5 times a day then try skipping 3 meals/day instead of one. This is beneficial especially if you are also doing calorie counting where you eat 1000 calories a day.

Intermittent fasting boosts your energy levels by forcing your body to burn fat as fuel, instead of the glucose stored in the liver and muscles. This is achieved by restricting how much you eat during the day. To start intermittent fasting, make it a clear rule that you will not eat for up to 16 hours out of the 24-hour cycle (e.g., from midnight until 4 am). Follow this rule for at least 3 days while taking note of how you feel after restricting eating time, and adjust as needed if there is no hunger or cravings present. Slow down your eating time at 9 pm and then slowly increase your eating time back to 12pm until it is back to your usual feeding routine.

Fasting also reduces the amount of insulin that is released, so it will reduce sugar cravings. It takes a month or two before your body adapts to this new way of using fat as fuel and hence less hunger pangs.

Fasting drinking is the most effective way to boost energy levels, but if you are not comfortable drinking during fasting hours, you can also take lemon and peppermint tea or infusion of fresh ginger and cinnamon to avoid sugar spikes. Hydrate yourself through water (one glass per hour works well), because it contains many important nutrients including electrolytes, which help with absorption and excretion of toxins.

Fasting also helps eliminate toxins that can cause chronic diseases, fatigue and weight gain. Toxins are stored in fat, so fasting encourages the body to burn fat as fuel instead of sugar.

How long you should fast depends on your body type and normal food intake. If you have a lot of body fat or feel heavy, try not eating for 16 hours at the beginning, then extend to 18 hours and later to 20 hours if 20 hours is still comfortable for your body. If you're already lean and active, try going longer without food – up to 24 hours.

If this is the first time you are trying intermittent fasting, start with an 8-hour period (e.g., 12 pm until 8 pm) and gradually increase to a 12-hour period (e.g., 12pm-8pm).

Incorporate foods that are rich in protein, low in carbs and good fats into your routine to maintain muscle mass, maximize fat burning and maintain energy levels throughout the day. Always include breakfast and lunch as these meals have been shown to be more satiating. If possible, try adding some exercise during fasting hours (e.g., a brisk 15-minute walk). Intermittent fasting is not suitable for people who are diabetic or on medicines that cause weight gain, so consult with your doctor before starting intermittent fasting if you have any of these conditions.

You will be more energetic when fasted and you will begin to see changes in your body after just a few weeks. With regular fasting days, you can also start getting used to skipping meals so that you can take the 8-hour period of eating as a treat rather than something to be normal.

It is difficult for most people who are used to 3 square meals a day and it is also hard for the body to adapt from using carbs as energy source to using fat stores instead, but intermittent fasting is one of the most effective ways for people who have difficulty maintaining a healthy weight or staying energetic throughout the day.

<u>Practical tips on intermittent fasting</u>

1. Breakfast is the most important meal of the day and eating it first thing in the morning aids weight loss and even prevents overeating at lunchtime.

2. Eat a protein-rich breakfast such as eggs, sausage or bacon for maximum fat burning and satiation.

3. While fasting, eat only one meal a day; don't eat in between and you will likely lose more weight than if you had just simply stayed on your regular diet regimen.

4. Identify your hunger triggers: know why you are hungry and learn how to satisfy it before it can take over your mind and cause over-eating throughout the day.

5. Eat only once or twice a day, but don't stay hungry between meals.

6. Take intermittent fasting seriously; if you do not eat enough to keep yourself awake, you will become tired and sleepy.

7. Follow a very high-calorie diet that is high in protein and reduces your consumption of carbohydrate-rich foods and simple sugars in order to maintain steady energy levels while following an intermittent fasting schedule.

8. Make sure that you drink at least 2 liters of water daily and take supplements for proper hydration during your fast.

9. Always follow proper fitness routines because exercise will help you burn more calories as well as keep you fit.

<u>How to manage cravings while intermittent fasting</u>

Just like everything else in life, intermittent fasting is one of those things with numerous advantages but has to be carefully managed. One of the main aspects to be aware of is that intermittent fasting can trigger cravings and sugar shocks, which may lead to a person wanting to eat something that they would not normally have as part of their diet. This chapter will discuss what you need to do if this does happen so you can get back into your fast as soon as possible and handle your cravings. All too often we go from one extreme dieting phase straight onto the next, never giving our bodies or minds time to adapt fully and recover from the previous phase.

What cravings are

First of all, when we talk about cravings, what we are talking about is the feeling you get in your gut that urges you to eat something (anything) that you would not usually eat. There are plenty of factors that can contribute to this feeling from lack of sleep to stress or even certain foods such as alcohol triggering a sugar rush (or crash). However, the most likely cause for most people is food. For some people this might be desserts or sweets; for others it might be carbs, fat, cheese and bread.

Why we get cravings

The reason we get cravings is that our bodies are constantly trying to maintain our energy levels. We don't move around the way we used to, eat the amount that we used to and our activity levels have decreased (along with weight loss). All these things do not leave much energy available for any other purpose. To compensate for this, there is a release of certain hormones such as adrenaline which act on your brain resulting in an urge to eat food that contains carbohydrates and protein. This is why you feel a craving for something sweet or salty--that provides the energy. The main reason that we are low on energy is because we are not eating enough. If we are not eating enough, then it is no surprise that our body and mind will start to send out signals to us about all the things that need to be done (e.g. "I am hungry; therefore, I need to eat").

HOW TO MANAGE CRAVINGS

The key to dealing with cravings is to know when the feeling is coming on and how to deal with it. It is possible that a craving may start even without any food present in your stomach. This can happen when you are stress, worried or experiencing other cravings such as wanting to chew on something. In this case, it means that the blood sugar levels are getting low and your body is telling you that you need energy.

STRATEGY #1 AVOID THE SUGAR RUSH

The best way to manage this type of craving is to not give yourself a sugar rush (energy crash) by eating something high calorie and high in carbohydrates. By doing this you will restore those energy levels that have been depleted by your fasting journey so far. This is why so many people will add some type of bread, rice or pasta in their diet during their intermittent fasts (often almost every day). This is the wrong way to deal with this craving because it will cause you to miss out on your daily calorie intake.

STRATEGY #2 DON'T GIVE INTO THE CRAVING

You need to understand that the idea of not giving into a craving is not about depriving yourself or faking positive thoughts. It is actually the exact opposite. When you are in a situation where you have an urge to eat, the most important thing to do is to focus on your breathing and eventually this will take away from any cravings you may be experiencing. Take a deep breath in through your nose and out through your mouth (a slow inhale and exhale). Another technique that can be useful is imagining relaxing places such as beaches, relaxing landscapes etc.

STRATEGY #3 DO NOT EAT UNTIL THE CRAVING PASSES

A good way to deal with cravings is to wait until the craving passes before you eat. This means you will be waiting as long as possible for it to pass, so much so that your body has suppressed all of your hunger signals and you are not actually even experiencing hunger any more. Some people find this a difficult concept to understand and may feel that they have nothing to worry about as they are already well on their way of losing weight by being on an intermittent fast. However, you have to understand the difference between craving and hunger.

If you are fasting and experience some type of craving such as wanting something sweet, then you need to allow your cravings to pass. If you can allow yourself to get past that craving by doing a series of breathing exercises or even listening to some music, then this is the time when those calories will be released from your body without any type of waste. This is the key concept behind intermittent fasting.

Once you have managed your cravings, it is important that you still eat a normal sized meal when it comes around--so that your body doesn't go into starvation mode trying to preserve your fat stores thinking that there is no food coming in (there will be).

STRATEGY #4 KEEP YOUR CRAVINGS IN PERSPECTIVE

Most of us tend to think that if we want something, then we should go and get it. This is how the majority of life works and seems like a logical approach. However, that is not the case. Instead, you need to keep things in perspective. A craving is only going to last for a short amount of time as it will eventually pass once your body has adjusted to your fasting journey so far. It may take several days or weeks for this to happen but it will happen at some point if you persevere with your dieting efforts. Remember that cravings are simply an indication that something is wrong (such as low energy levels). It is up to you to fix the underlying issue, rather than simply doing something that will satisfy that craving in the short term.

STRATEGY #5 DO NOT KEEP FOOD AROUND THE HOUSE

There is no point in having a jar of biscuits or some type of junk food in your cupboard if you are going to be fasting on a regular basis. Rather than having these types of things readily available for you when you want them, it is much better to not have them at all. If they are not there then there is nothing for you to eat and this will help with coping with cravings too. Your body will get used to eating smaller meals and eventually won't even think about wanting anything else.

STRATEGY #6 EAT A HEALTHY DIET

When you are exercising on a regular basis then you are going to need to ensure that your body has the appropriate energy levels in order to perform at its best. The most effective way to do this is by eating meals that contain carbohydrates such as pasta, rice, vegetables and rice. You should also include some type of protein in each meal such as fish or meat, which will provide your body with the building blocks that it needs in order to have strong muscles and great determination during your exercise regime.

If it is possible for you to drink milk, then this is ideal as it contains lots of carbohydrates too.

<u>Mistakes to avoid</u>

#1 Not having a plan in place

Intermittent fasting isn't a free-for-all diet. It can take some finesse and careful planning if you want the process to be successful. For example, what you eat the day before and after a fast can have a big impact on your success. The biggest mistake that intermittent fasters make is not planning out what they're going to eat, when and how much. Simply going without eating for a period of time doesn't make for an effective intermittent fasting plan if you don't know what you're doing.

#2 Drinking too many fluids

Just because you're not eating anything doesn't mean that you should drink as much as you want. A lot of people think they have to drink more when they do intermittent fasting- that isn't true at all! You only need to drink when it feels natural for your body. If you feel thirsty, then drink- but only drink as much as your body tells you to.

#3 Fasting too long

Intermittent fasting is not for everyone. Some people do fine with intermittent fasting while others just can't handle it. If you're an active person or if you have a job that requires a lot of focus and energy, then it might not be the best option for you. Most people don't realize this and give intermittent fasting a try anyway…only to find themselves discouraged and disappointed in the results.

#4 Drinking too many artificial energy drinks and powders

For some people, having an artificial boost while they're on a fast will help. For others, this can cause them to feel even more fatigued and irritable. You should make sure that you're fully hydrated before you break your fast and consume energy drinks or powders. And if you find yourself cheating or binging when breaking your fast, then these drinks are not for you!

#5 Skipping breakfast

Intermittent fasting is a lot easier for most people when they start the day off with a healthy breakfast. If you skip breakfast or wait too long to eat in the morning, then you're going to struggle with your fast. Your body needs fuel when fasting so make sure that you have a good breakfast each morning before starting your fast.

#6 Eating too much during your feeding periods

Some people try to "get their money's worth" when they break their fast. Some people binge because they think they need to consume as much as possible during the feeding period. That's not true at all! You only need an amount of food that will keep your body at a fasting state. You don't need to stuff yourself or overdo it.

#7 Not drinking enough water

When you stop eating, your body is going through a process of cleansing and resetting itself. Part of this process is going to require more fluids than you normally consume. It's important to stay well hydrated throughout the day so your body will cleanse efficiently and quickly. If you're not properly hydrated, then your body has to work even harder to get rid of all those toxins that are floating around in your bloodstream and organs.

#8 Forgetting about vitamins and minerals

You might be surprised by how much more vitamins and minerals you need while fasting. If you're not getting enough of these important nutrients, then your body won't function properly. You need to make sure that you're getting a good amount of vitamins and minerals while you're fasting.

#9 Going longer than intended

Many people who try intermittent fasting decide that it isn't for them after they push the envelope during a fast. If you want to get the most out of intermittent fasting, then it needs to be done right for it to work effectively.

Intermittent fasting for Type 2 Diabetes

This chapter explains how intermittent fasting can be used to reduce the risk of developing Type 2 Diabetes and reverse it in those who already have it. It will also go over what kind of foods are eaten while intermittent fasting and what kind of benefits you can expect from intermittent fasting with regards to reducing the risk for Type 2 diabetes and reversing it. For those looking to get started or want some help figuring out what diet they should be on this chapter has a fourth part that breaks down the best diet strategies for Type 2 Diabetes.

Type 2 Diabetes is a condition in which the body does not properly use insulin. It is also referred to as adult-onset diabetes, hyperglycemia, and non-insulin-dependent diabetes mellitus (NIDDM). Type 2 Diabetes has over 250 million sufferers worldwide and usually starts later in life between the ages of 40 and 60 years old. In the US alone there are 20 million people suffering from Type 2 Diabetes.

The prevalence of Type 2 Diabetes is increasing from both the increased weight in the population combined with the rise in the number of obese and overweight people. The obesity epidemic is continuing to spread around the world and there are hopes that it will start to level off by 2025 through governmental measures of fighting this problem.

What Diet Should Be Followed While Intermittent Fasting?

What kind of diet should be followed while intermittent fasting? Now that you understand what intermittent fasting is and why it is so beneficial, you might want to know how you can apply this information to help fight off or get rid of your Type 2 Diabetes.

If you are looking to get started with intermittent fasting, make sure you find a diet that is expected to be most beneficial for your condition and health in general. While it does not matter what type of food you eat in regards to the intermittent fasting schedule, it would be a good idea to have a diet that has healthy fats, vegetables, and plant-based foods.

These are some of the foods I recommend to start off with:

- Bone Broth: Bone broth is really good for you as it boosts up your immunity and helps you feel better. It also has anti-inflammatory properties which is why I recommended it to start off with because the immune system will need all the help it can get from fighting off inflammation from the inflammation that is caused by Chronic Fatigue Syndrome.

- Healthy Fats: High in Omega 3's and 6's, they are vital if you have Chronic Fatigue Syndrome because these two fatty acids help fight diseases such as cancer, Alzheimer's disease, or even diabetes by reducing inflammation. As I mentioned earlier in this chapter, make sure you have a diet high in vegetables and other fruits.

- Veggies: Make sure you eat a lot of the following vegetables: cucumbers, bell peppers, celery, kale, tomatoes, broccoli, and carrots. These are all fantastic sources of vitamin C and antioxidants along with being loaded with a host of anti-inflammatory vitamins that can lower your overall risk for Type 2 Diabetes: vitamin A (beta-carotene) , vitamin K (folate) , C (ascorbic acid), folate , and E .

- Fiber: Fiber is the only type of carbohydrate that has been linked to a reduced risk of Type 2 Diabetes.

When starting out with intermittent fasting, you can gradually transition into it instead of just going on a low-calorie diet. For example, if your calorie intake for the day is around 2,000 calories a day, you can start out by reducing your intake to 1,500 calories.

If you decide to do this, it will be harder to reduce your weight but the benefits of intermittent fasting are still present along with reducing your insulin resistance that could lead to Type 2 Diabetes or even Pre-Diabetes.

Combating Diabetes with the 5:2 intermittent fasting diet

This is another diet that can be considered along with intermittent fasting when it comes to fighting off or reversing Type 2 Diabetes. It is known as the 5:2 intermittent fasting diet and basically involves eating 500 calories at 5 a.m. and 2 p.m. This is great for people who can't always eat at those times because of work or other commitments but also good for those who just don't want to fast because they have to work around their time schedule and can only fast for one day out of the week that they are on intermittent fasting.

The benefits of this kind of diet are still present by reducing your insulin resistance as well as improving your overall health, weight management, and most importantly Blood Sugar Levels.

One may wonder if this diet is sustainable or not but honestly it is. I know people who are doing this diet and have been able to support themselves with this kind of schedule. It can be done without even having to buy any special foods and you only need two breakfast foods and two comfort foods for the rest of the week. See Dan Buettner's interview on eating with intermittent fasting for a more detailed look at how he started doing it:

Fasting plays a pivotal role in regaining control over one's health, insulin receptors, and metabolism. With the proper guidance, people can lose body weight and reverse diabetes reversal.

CHAPTER 5: INTERMITTENT FASTING AND EXERCISE

Working out while intermittent fasting can be a little complicated, but there are ways to make it easier. Women over 50 years old may want to incorporate exercise with intermittent fasting. What's the best way for women over 50 to combine exercise with intermittent fasting?

The key is not to eat too much after working out. It is not necessary to eat as soon as you finish exercising, wait at least a couple hours and then make your meal small and light. For example, if you have worked out in the morning - wait until about noon or later for your meal and include some protein and vegetables in it. You may want to avoid eating too many fibrous foods that can cause digestive issues such as gas or bloating during a workout session. It is possible to do intermittent fasting without exercise, but the combination is especially beneficial for women over 50 years old. When you work out while intermittent fasting your body burns more calories and fat. This will help you lose weight and keep it off, especially if you incorporate exercise with intermittent fasting on a regular basis.

Walking or hiking is a great way to get some exercise in while still eating only one meal per day. If you walk at a brisk pace, you can burn as many as 50 calories per 3-4 miles. Walking or hiking should be done for at least 30 minutes to be effective in burning fat and keeping the weight off. (36 calories per mile for walking).

When you combine intermittent fasting with exercise, the benefits can be substantial. Intermittent fasting will help you lose weight by burning more fat. It can also help you get leaner if you use exercise with intermittent fasting on a regular basis as it will help to keep your metabolism up and burn even more calories. There are many reports of women doing intermittent fasting and exercising on a regular basis and losing several pounds in just a short period of time.

One great thing about intermittent fasting is that it doesn't have to hurt your workout program like some fad diets do. When you fast, there are no negative side effects that interfere with your workout program such as other fad diets cause. With intermittent fasting you can eat throughout the day and not have to worry about it interfering with your workouts.

Cardio

There are many benefits of cardio exercise, but for women over 50 years old there are also some specific benefits associated with cardio exercise. Women over 50 years old who do cardio exercise can improve their cholesterol levels. This is because when you burn fat while doing cardio, it is released into the blood stream where it attaches to certain proteins called apoproteins and then is taken back out of the blood stream into the liver where it is used as an energy source for the body. This can help your cholesterol levels if you do cardio exercise and intermittent fasting.

Cardio exercise helps reduce the risk of heart disease and stroke. When women over 50 years old do cardio exercise, it keeps their cardiovascular system strong, which will help prevent heart disease and stroke. Women over 50 years old who have a healthy lifestyle can play an important role in the prevention of heart disease and stroke.

CARDIO EXERCISE 1: JUMPING

When you jump with your whole body, your muscles work harder as they are used to the stress which results in higher metabolism. Your muscles will become stronger and more toned as you move your body more often during the day during cardio exercise such as running or walking. You can work up to doing cardio exercise for 30 minutes, several times per week.

CARDIO EXERCISE 2: RUNNING/JOGGING

Running or jogging is one of the best cardio exercises and is excellent for women over 50 years old who do no other kinds of exercise. Running or jogging may not be necessary for younger women who are only in their 20s and 30s, but if you are over 50 years old it is a great way to keep your body fit and healthy. You will burn more calories during the run, so you will have more energy throughout the day. You can increase the amount of time you run depending upon how much time you have available due to work schedule or other responsibilities that need to be met.

It is very important for women over 50 years old to stay active and exercise. If you don't, your body will begin to shut down faster. You need to do cardio exercise 2 - 3 times per week for optimal results.

When you combine cardio exercise with intermittent fasting, particularly during the morning hours, it will help you lose weight and keep it off as your body burns more fat with the combination. The fat that is burned by the combination usually isn't stored in another place but is actually released into your blood stream where it attaches to various proteins and then is taken back out of your body for use as an energy source during normal operation of your body system.

Weight Training

Women over 50 can also benefit from the improved bone health that comes from weight training. It also helps you build lean muscle tissue. This will help you burn more calories throughout the day.

Weight lifting is very important for women over 50 years old as this is a time when your body begins to deteriorate. The weight lifting you do helps build and repair your muscles, which is an important part of having a healthy body in your fifties. It is also very important that you maintain a healthy diet while doing weight lifting, as an imbalanced diet can slow down the effectiveness of weight training or even result in negative side effects such as sore joints or muscles, headaches and other discomforts.

Weight lifting can be done several times per week for 30 minutes. If you are doing weight lifting and cardio exercise 2 - 3 times per week, it will be beneficial to do this in the morning to start your day off as this will get your metabolism going and improve your body's overall health. Women over 50 years old should have no problem losing weight due to weight lifting and working out.

You can also take advantage of free weights at home or visit a gym for a strength training class. A good strength training routine for women over 50 years old consists of 4 sets of 10 - 12 repetitions with 1 minute rest between each set.

Weight training will help you keep a healthy weight and improve your metabolism. You should do strength training one to two times per week for 30 minutes to 45 minutes.

<u>Exercises that you can do at home</u>

For women who don't have the time to go to the gym, you can do a lot of exercises at home and still be able to lose weight.

1. Yoga

Yoga is a good one for women over 50 years old as it helps with flexibility. Yoga can help you in other ways, such as improving your sleep. If you need more energy throughout the day, try doing yoga during the morning hours instead of doing cardio exercise first thing in the morning. Some aerobic exercises can actually be counterproductive if they are done too soon after eating breakfast.

You can do yoga at home by following a DVD. Yoga can be done in the morning or evening. For women over 50, Yoga is a good option that will help you lose weight and stay healthy.

2. Calisthenics

Calisthenics is ideal for women over 50 years old who want to lose weight fast. This refers to exercises such as push-ups, pull-ups, sit-ups and squats that can be done without any equipment. Calisthenics is very simple to do at home and can help you lose weight quite quickly. The great thing about calisthenics is that it doesn't take up much time. You can do calisthenics in the morning, evening or even at night before you go to bed.

3. Dance

Dancing can also be a good option for women over 50 years old who don't have a lot of time because it burns calories and is fun to do. Dancing does not only refer to ballroom dancing but any type of dance you might enjoy doing. It can help you with balance, flexibility and getting more exercise into your day.

It is not necessary to be a professional to do so. You can just pick up a dance class at the community gym or borrow one of your friend's classes from time to time. If you feel you are not getting enough exercise, you can try different types of dance such as salsa, waltz and tango.

4. Aerobics

Aerobics refers to an aerobic exercise routine that involves rhythmic movements performed with the use of our own body weight and muscle power in order to burn calories. The benefits of aerobics are improved posture, body tone, better cardiovascular health and increased flexibility and energy levels.

Chapter 6: Intermittent Fasting to Regain Youthfulness

BODY COMPOSITION CHANGE

In chapter five it was mentioned that muscle tissue is burned from the workout while fat tissue is stored as energy for the body. If you have been exercising for a long time it is possible that your body composition has changed. In other words, if you have been exercising for a long time your muscles might have become larger and more toned than they were when you started. Women over 50 years old are often the most likely to have this type of change.

You can easily see this happen when you lose muscle definition when you start exercising again. If you start exercising again while you still have a lot of muscle tone, it is very easy to get discouraged and stop exercising because your muscles are no longer shaped into the shape they were in when you first started.

This can be caused by a number of reasons, including:

1. Your metabolism has slowed down: If your metabolism has slowed down as you get older it is possible that your body just isn't burning fat during exercise at the same rate as it used to when you were younger.

2. Your exercise routine is no longer effective: If you have been exercising the same way for a long time and don't change it up from time to time, your exercise routine can become ineffective over time. The reason for this is that your body will become accustomed to doing the same exercises repeatedly. Your body will get used to the certain

movements and no longer realize that they are needing to use more energy than before.

3. You are doing too much: It is possible that you are exercising too much and your body just doesn't have the energy it needs to keep up.

4. Your body is not getting enough nutrients: If your body is not getting enough nutrients, it will be less able to burn fat during exercise.

It is important to keep in mind that doing an exercise routine for a long period of time will inevitably cause some changes in your body composition. The key is to always keep a positive attitude and change your exercise routine from time to time so that you don't get bored out of exercising all together.

Try the following tips in order to help regain your youthful appearance:

1. Remember that it's normal for your muscles to get smaller than they were when you first started exercising. Just because your muscles are not as large as they used to be does not mean that you should give up on exercising altogether.

2. Be sure to vary the exercises you do so that your body does not become accustomed to doing the same exercises over and over again.

3. Try exercising in a different way than you have been doing. For example, if you have been going to the gym and using weights, try going for a walk instead or swimming laps in the pool at your local gym. This will help your body become more flexible and toned too!

4. Try changing up the time of day when you exercise throughout the week as well so that you don't get bored out of it altogether.

5. Try doing your exercises when you're not at peak levels of energy. This will help you get through exercising more consistently.

6. Try exercising when your energy levels are higher so that you don't have to rely on your body's natural ability to burn fat while exercising.

7. If possible, try working out at the same time as someone else so you will get some encouragement and motivation while you are working out with others.

8. Try working out during the morning hours if you can. Evening exercise is still very important, but if you can do your exercise during the morning hours your exercise will be more effective and your body will not get so bored of exercising.

When you hit the big five-oh, it's sometimes hard to accept that you are getting older. It is easy to feel disappointed when you feel like your body is getting older as well and no matter how much exercise or healthy eating you do, your body just isn't what it used to be.

Because it's a natural process for our bodies to deteriorate as we get older, there really isn't anything we can do about it. However, there are things that women over 50 should start doing in order to maintain their youthful appearance without resorting to plastic surgery or other mainstream methods.

There are many ways women over 50 can look and feel younger than ever before without spending tons of money on expensive products or procedures. Here are just a few tips to help you look more youthful and stay healthy:

1. Get up earlier throughout the week: By getting up before your normal bed time, your body will be more alert for the day as well as more active during the day. This will help you get moving during the day as well as burn extra calories.

2. Start including some exercise in your daily lifestyle: If you really can't find the energy to exercise throughout the week, try doing a small workout at home such as yoga, playing tennis or riding a stationary bike every now and again throughout the week to help combat that sluggish feeling you might be feeling throughout the day!

3. Eat more fruits and vegetables: Fruits and vegetables are rich in nutrients that can help you stay healthy. They also have the added benefit of helping you lose weight if you are looking to reduce your overall body mass.

4. Try drinking green tea: Green tea is a great way to fight off the harmful free radicals that promote aging while helping improve your health overall.

5. Avoid drinking too much alcohol: Although we all love a good glass of wine once in a while, it is important to not over indulge in this habit as it can cause inflammation throughout your entire body as well as damage blood vessels. Excessive alcohol consumption can also lead to reduced brain function which causes grey hair and wrinkles!

6. Try not to smoke: Smoking can cause many health conditions such as high blood pressure, heart disease and lung cancer so it is best to avoid this habit if you can.

7. Try doing some of these exercises throughout the day:

- Yoga: Yoga is great for helping strengthen your bones and muscles while making your body more flexible.

- Aerobics: If you have been leading a sedentary lifestyle, or just don't feel like exercising, try taking up a formal cardio routine such as jogging or swimming every now and again throughout the week.

8. Avoid eating too much sodium: Sodium can cause fluid retention in your body and make you puffier than normal so it is important to follow a low level of sodium diet when you can.

9. Eat foods that are rich in estrogen: Beans, soy, seeds and flax all have estrogen in them which will help your body stay healthy while also helping to reduce the effects of menopause as well.

10. Try to drink one or two glasses of red wine when you feel like you need it: Red wine is a good source of antioxidants which help fight various conditions such as heart disease, cancer and skin problems. It is also a great source of nutrients such as magnesium which helps your heart beat more regularly.

11. If you are over 50, try taking vitamin E: Vitamin E can help reduce the signs of aging in your skin and prevent sun damage along with other common health problems.

CHAPTER 7: INTERMITTENT FASTING LIFESTYLE

*Everything comes to pass;
nothing comes to stay-Mathew
Flickstine*

The idea behind intermittent fasting is that if you give your digestive system a break, it won't function as hard and your body will be more efficient at breaking down food into energy. There are many benefits to intermittent fasting such as losing weight, improving overall health or just making your life easier in general.

If you want to try this type of lifestyle but aren't sure where to start, here are some tips on how to make intermittent fasting easier:

1. Make sure you have a good eating schedule. The idea behind intermittent fasting is that your body will break down food more efficiently if you give it a break, so make sure you don't eat for 8 hours every day. Try doing this for 5 days and record how much weight you lose by following this guide.

2. Try to maintain the same amount of sleep each night: Intermittent fasting can increase your metabolism in order to help burn calories throughout the day, so make sure you are getting good quality sleep every night as this will help too!

3. Don't eat right before bed: Make sure that you are not eating anything around 2 hours before bedtime. If you still have an appetite, drink a glass of water with some lemon juice in it to curb your appetite.

4. Wake up 1 hour earlier than usual: This will help stimulate your metabolism and give your body the energy it needs for the day.

5. Try to do some kind of exercise every day: Intermittent fasting is often conducted in conjunction with other

healthful lifestyle choices such as exercising more often, drinking more water and eating healthy foods so make sure you don't miss out on these benefits as well by adding exercise into your daily lifestyle once you start doing intermittent fasting!

Although it is possible to lose weight on nearly any diet, a healthy diet is necessary if you want to maintain your youthful appearance and health. The goal of a healthy diet is to provide your body with the nutrients it needs while ensuring that you're not consuming too many calories and avoiding foods that are bad for your health. It's possible to lose weight without having to do any exercise at all. You can boost your metabolism naturally by doing simple things such as:

1. Start improving your eating habits

If you have been eating the same way for a long time, you will most likely gain weight unless you change things around. Learn to eat more slowly, chew your food thoroughly and be conscious of all the calories that you eat. Make sure to eat 3 balanced meals a day and avoid to eating too much junk food. Be sure to eat all your vitamins and minerals

Make sure you are getting all the basic nutrients your body needs by including a variety of fruits, vegetables, whole grains and lean proteins in your diet.

2. Be active

When you don't exercise, your body needs to produce more energy from the food you eat to maintain its normal functions. This means that you can lose weight without having to exercise if you eat a healthy diet and get a good amount of exercise throughout your everyday life.

3. Drink water

The average person should be drinking 2 liters of water daily in order for their bodies to function properly and stay healthy without becoming dehydrated or losing too much fluid. It is also important that the water you drink is fresh so it can also prevent diseases such as heart disease, kidney disease and bladder infections.

4. Maintain your weight

Being overweight puts extra stress on your body and can lead to a lot of other health problems such as heart disease and cancer. Keeping yourself at a healthy weight will help you maintain your youthful appearance while also reducing the risk of heart disease and keeping your body functioning correctly.

5. Exercise regularly

If you want to lose weight without worrying about exercising, it is important that you start getting active throughout the day instead! It is also important to do some sort of exercise daily as well in order to keep your body toned.

6. Stay away from harmful substances

Avoid drinking excessive amounts of alcohol and avoid smoking cigarettes as these are both dangerous for your overall health in terms of damaged organs, cancer and lung diseases. Although they are enjoyable in moderation, it is important to realize that too much can be bad for your body!

7. Take supplements

Taking supplements will help you get all the essential vitamins and minerals that your body needs while ensuring that you are completely healthy and positive. You should start taking any supplements at least 2 weeks before you plan to stop working out as your body will have a lot of adjusting to do.

8. Try a new diet

If you think that your current diet might not be healthy for you and you aren't losing any weight, try to find a healthy alternative that appeals to your taste buds. A popular diet is the Paleo Diet which advocates eating like our caveman ancestors. The diet is based around real food and has many benefits as it is very low in sugar, cholesterol and refined foods.

9. Water:

Drinking water is vital as it helps to flush your body out and keep you hydrated (it can also help your skin as well!).

10. Avoid the wrong foods

Although it is sometimes difficult, try to avoid foods that are not good for you as this will greatly improve your health and help you lose weight more easily!

This section will cover some advice for grocery shopping when you are on an intermittent fasting diet as well as what foods to eat during this diet with plenty of information to help you out with the right training programs and meal plans for your body type.

Before we look at the different options for getting healthy food, we need to ask ourselves why it is so important that you are eating healthy. Weight loss is not a big deal if it isn't for health reasons. We all have been told that being well-nourished gives your immune system a boost, boosts metabolism and helps to keep weight off. If your body is constantly craving food, it's hard to lose weight by cutting calories down.

vegetables

The first thing to bear in mind is that you need to be including a lot of vegetables

into your diet. These are the building blocks for everything else. You will also notice that making a smoothie, juicing or eating raw vegetables are great ways to get all the nutrients you need and still consume all the vitamins, minerals and enzymes. Buy vegetables rich I vitamins A, B and C as these will boost your immune system and help you stay alert during the day. Another great benefit of eating vegetables is that they are low in calories, high in fiber and can fill you up quickly.

Vegetable's shopping list

-Chard (avoid Swiss chard as it is very high in calories and can cause bloating)

– Cucumbers (the thinner ones are best)

– Eggplant

– Lettuce (romaine, butter or dark green varieties work best for this meal)

-Romaine lettuce hearts

-Mushrooms

-Onions (red onions are the best.

Avoid onions if you are a diabetic)

– Radishes (good for blood circulation and digestion)

– Spinach (a great source of iron and calcium. Try to buy fresh spinach when possible as it is higher in nutrients)

Fruits

Next, try to up your fruit intake to at least two or three servings per day. Fruit is a natural source of fructose which helps to keep your metabolism running, keep your blood sugar levels up and makes you feel full as well. The other great thing about fruit is that it is so full of vitamins, minerals and antioxidants. Apples are one of the highest in vitamin C which can help you to fight off viruses as well as increase your body's immunity.

Avoid eating fruit every day as it is easy to exceed your daily calorie count by doing this. Make sure you get a variety of colors by choosing from oranges, berries, apples, peaches or pears.

Fruit's shopping list

-Apples (red are the best. If you have a sensitive stomach, only eat one. They are also a good source of soluble fiber which can lower cholesterol and reduce the risk of heart disease.)

-Apricots (a good source of vitamin A and D along with antioxidants)

– Bananas (good for heart health, perfect for exercise recovery or eaten before bed)

– Blackberries (full of antioxidants, iron and calcium)

– Blueberries (good for improving memory and concentration levels. Can also increase your body's immunity to cancer as well as high levels of antioxidants.

– Cantaloupe (full of antioxidants, a good source of nutrients and is perfect for cleansing the body)

– Clementine's (small and easy to pack up when traveling. Another citrus fruit that is full of nutrients, antioxidants and vitamin C)

– Figs (good for curing constipation as it has a lot of fiber as well as being high in calcium and antioxidants)

– Grapefruit (can help to lower cholesterol but can also cause some side effects such as indigestion when eaten on an empty stomach. Avoid refined grapefruits, eat organic if possible.

– Grapes (a great source of antioxidants and other nutrients)

– Honeydew melon (good for supplying energy, can also help you to lose weight and lowers cholesterol)

– Kiwi (high in fiber, vitamin C and a good source of potassium)

– Mango (full of antioxidants, helps to lower cholesterol and is full of vitamins)

– Nectarines (another good fruit for lowering cholesterol as well as another good source of vitamins A and C.)

-Oranges (high in fiber, contains a lot of vitamin C. Can help to lower cholesterol, is good for digestion and improves your skin's appearance too.)

-Papaya (rich in enzymes as well as being full of vitamins and antioxidants)

– Peaches (high in vitamins A, C and fiber. Can help to lower cholesterol levels, improve heart health

and protect against cancer)

– Pears (good for heart health, helps to prevent stomach ulcers and can help you to lose weight if eaten before bedtime)

– Pineapple (rich in manganese which helps with bone strength as well as a powerful digestive enzyme brome line which can be helpful if you are suffering from indigestion.

– Plums (good for skin, can help to lower cholesterol and improve heart health)

– Watermelon (high in fiber, can help to prevent diabetes as well as helping with digestion)

Fats

Fat is very important because it helps to keep your body healthy. It also keeps you feeling full for longer and keeps you feeling energized throughout the day.

Egg yolks are one of the best sources of fat as well as a source of protein and omega-3 fatty acids that will help keep your skin young. Salmon makes a great snack in moderation while other fatty fish such as tuna, mackerel, sardines and herring can be eaten in small amounts when you want some extra protein in your diet. Cottage cheese, avocado -which contains vitamin E- and nuts are also good for adding some extra fat to your diet too.

Fat's shopping list

-Avocados

– Cheese (full fat or vegetarian I'm certain is good for fat loss) – Dairy products (try to avoid the skimmed milk as it is high in sugar)

– Full-fat yogurts

– Ghee (good for your heart and skin) – Halibut

– Mackerel (rich in omega 3 fatty acids. Can be a little messy to prepare but it is very good for your skin, aids in digestion and helps you lose weight.

Nuts

Nuts are a great source of healthy fats which will help you to lose weight while also sustaining energy throughout the day. Nuts are also amazing for their protein content which is great for building up muscle while helping you to make new muscle tissues as well. Women should be eating around 3–4oz per day, while men should be eating 6–8oz per day. Nuts can be a little more expensive than the other foods on the list but if you buy in bulk, it will last a long time.

Nut's shopping list

– Macadamias (good for heart health and can lower acidity levels)

– Almonds (very high in vitamin E and fiber. Can be good for lowering cholesterol, improve heart health

and help to cleanse the body)

– Pine nuts

– Hazelnuts (can aid in digestion, can help you to lose weight and can lower cholesterol levels) – Walnuts (high in omega-3 fatty acids which are essential for a healthy heart while also helping you to lose weight)

CHAPTER 8: DETOXING YOUR BODY THROUGH INTERMITTENT FASTING

DETOX your mind, body, AND your contact list.
-Supa Nova Slom

Detox

Detox refers to the act of ridding your body of toxic substances. In the last year or two, we've been hearing a lot about detoxing as a way to improve our health. We're told that we should clean out our livers and kidneys, or eat foods that will help us rid our bodies of toxins.

Toxins

These are substances that we don't need and that can be harmful to our bodies. When people talk about toxins in our environment, they're usually talking about pollution in the air, water, or the soil. We also have a lot of chemicals in our food supply and even in some of the things we use all day long.

The detox process

Our bodies have ways of getting rid of extra wastes that we ingest or produce. The liver is the organ that's in charge of breaking down and deactivating substances that come into our bodies. The liver produces bile, which is stored in the gallbladder until it's ready to be released into the small intestine. Bile contains enzymes, which help to break down fats in the food we eat. Then a substance called glucuronic acid helps to neutralize toxins so they can be excreted by the kidneys and eliminated from our bodies through urine or feces.

Detox programs are designed to give your body a break from the usual processes that break down and eliminate toxins. For example, you might choose to fast once a year for several days so that your body can focus on getting rid of the toxins that have built up over time. Some people use herbs or other substances during this kind of fast.

The purpose behind an intermittent fasting program is to take your body out of its routine and make it work harder to eliminate wastes and cleanse itself naturally, without using food and water as a crutch.

While there are different ways to detox and it's impossible to say which is best for you, intermittent fasting is one option that can be done by anyone at any age. Intermittent fasting (IF) involves eating only during certain times of the day with periods of abstaining from food in between. What goes against what many people believe: IF might actually be easier on your digestive system than eating three or four meals every day.

One reason so many people are drawn to intermittent fasting is that it can help improve health. Long-term fasting reduces the risk of heart disease, diabetes, and cancer. Plus, eating less food and losing weight can burn more fat for you. If your goal is to improve your health, reducing your body fat percentage might be a big part of the plan.

Detox and the female body

When it comes to health, women are at a disadvantage. That's because they tend to have more body fat than men do. There is also some evidence that women's bodies are less able to get rid of toxins than men's bodies are, and that this is even more likely if you're overweight. Plus, if you're on birth control pills or have gone through menopause and are no longer producing eggs, your estrogen levels may be lower than they were when you were younger.

Women's bodies have certain health issues that would benefit from a natural detox like intermittent fasting or cleansing herbal teas. As a woman ages, her levels of estrogen, progesterone and testosterone begin to decline naturally. This is why we see signs of aging well before menopause. Our bodies are less able to produce certain hormones that ensure we feel and look healthy in the later years.

Estrogen helps to keep our bodies fit and active. It regulates the development of the body's tissues and also helps control how our cells divide and grow. For women it promotes heart health, growth, blood health, keeps skin smooth and hair shiny while regulating menstrual cycles to keep one step ahead of PMS symptoms like bloating caused by hormones fluctuating in the body.

In menopause the body's estrogen levels significantly drop as it begins to prepare for menopause. This results in unpleasant symptoms such as hot flashes, night sweats, insomnia and mood swings. During this time the body requires more nutrients and minerals which are supplied by a healthy diet.

If you follow intermittent fasting you may encounter fewer hot flashes since your body's ability to burn fat will increase when it isn't constantly digesting food. Reducing the amount of food you eat will also help decrease bloating and water retention. By following IF you can go about your daily routine without sweating excessively or having to change your wardrobe every day from being swollen and feeling feverish from water retention.

Although toxins aren't the only thing that can be harmful to our bodies, they are a major factor in many women's health problems. It's important to note that hormones and genetics play a role as well. There is no question about the fact that it is easier for women to get sick and have health issues than it is for men.

Women and men are not necessarily designed differently in terms of detoxing, although at times we may need extra help to get rid of these toxins. If you're experiencing toxin-related health issues, or if you think that your body may benefit from a natural detox, consider IF as a healthy alternative to eating three times a day.

<u>Why you should consider intermittent fasting for detox</u>

1. Detoxing rejuvenates your body

Every year more and more people turn to detoxing for better health. There is a growing trend toward using natural and effective methods like eating a healthy diet and going on periodic "cleanses" of sorts. In addition, there are many popular "detox diets" out there today, like green juice cleanses or specific herbs used to help your body detoxify itself.

Once you get your body back to its natural state, you will feel more energized, less bloated, less anxious and just happier overall. As you cleanse your system of harmful toxins, you will also find that your skin looks clearer and healthier than ever before. Plus, the added bonus is that it is inexpensive!

2. Detoxing makes your body stronger

One of the best ways to detox your body is through intermittent fasting. By eating smaller meals throughout the day, you are breaking down food so that your body has more energy to burn. By fasting at least once in a while, you will also be giving your immune system a boost. Your overall health and wellbeing will greatly improve as a result of doing this.

3. Detoxing gives you more energy

We know that diet plays a huge role in the amount of energy that we have all day long, but does it also make you feel energetic? Research has shown that eating foods high in sugar will cause you to feel less energetic than if you ate whole fresh foods instead.

During an intermittent fasting detox, you can eat as many fruits and vegetables as you want. This is a great way to get your daily recommended servings of fruits and vegetables, which are high in vitamins and minerals to give you more energy during the day.

When you are in a fasted state, your body is more efficient at using food for energy which results in heightened energy levels. So, if you want to be able to get through a hectic day, drinking plenty of water while you are fasting will help so that you are able to stay on top of things without getting tired. 8. Detoxing helps relieve nausea and headaches

Drinking lots of water while fasting gets rid of the toxins from your body that could be contributing to headaches and nausea so it is important to keep drinking water when you go through a fast!

4. Detoxing helps fight disease

In addition to helping lower your risk of developing heart disease, cancer or diabetes, it has also been shown that cleansing the body with fasting can have anti-aging effects on cells. This means that when we cleanse our bodies with fasting on a consistent basis we may live longer, healthier lives.

5. Detoxing helps you sleep better

If your goal is to get a good night's rest, it is important to do everything in your power to make sure that you are rested and ready for the day ahead. One way that can ensure a good night's rest is through a detox. When you cleanse your body on a regular basis, you will find that you will sleep better than ever before.

6. Detoxing gives better skin

One of the side effects of going through an extended period of fasting is that it will give healthy glowing skin without even any makeup. By ridding yourself of toxins, pimples and blemishes are cleared out too so it results in having healthier skin than ever before!

<u>How to improve your body's detox mechanism</u>

There are several ways to give your body a detox, but I believe that the simplest way is to have a fasting regimen. Starving your body does makes it detoxify naturally. However, this is not always enough for your liver to fully heal and flush out the toxins. In order to do a full body detox, you need to boost your body's natural immune system by consuming food that is packed with antioxidants.

Foods like berries, blueberries, green tea and cruciferous vegetables can boost the immune system to help get your body detoxifying throughout the entire year. Antioxidants also work to protect your cells from free radicals which can cause damage to DNA and other cell components. Although detoxification is a naturally occurring process in the body, a full body detox is important at certain stages of life such as during pregnancy or when ill.

Consider adding into your diet:

Believe it or not, your natural ability to detoxify may substantially deteriorate with age. Regardless of whether or not you eat processed foods or not, you may still need some extra help with detoxing between meals especially since you only need small amounts of food at a time.

Be sure to include raw vegetables and fruits in your diet starting the day after you eat a meal. You can also add some herbs like red clover which helps the liver work at a better rate. When you have a fasting detox, you will need to drink more water throughout the day but this is recommended for any type of detox.

Some of the best ideas that I've heard on how to improve your body's ability to detoxify includes adding in some herbs into your diet or taking supplements with activated charcoal, wheatgrass and acai berries.

Signs that you need to cleanse your system by fasting for a day or two

1. You get sick with a cold, stomach flu or sinus irritation frequently

Colds, flus and the common cold can all be caused by viruses that are generally causing a severe immune system response. If you are having trouble with these kinds of symptoms, it could be a sign that your immune system has been compromised, possibly due to the toxins that you do not eliminate properly. During and after a fast, it is important to supplement your diet with whatever vitamins and minerals that you need to re-establish your immune system.

2. You have skin problems like acne, chapped lips or any kind of dry skin

Dry skin can be a sign of inflammation which can be caused by a number of things like systemic inflammation from stress, exercise or poor diet. These kinds of conditions are easy to treat if you know the right foods to eat for relief from dryness. The best food to eat for healing dry skin is raw blueberries.

In addition, you can add 5-10 drops of frankincense essential oil into your bath water to stimulate collagen production so that dryness is alleviated. Another food that you should be drinking more of is coconut water. This natural supplement to add in your diet may help to improve moisture levels in the skin.

3. You have trouble with digestion (such as bloating).

There are a lot of foods that can cause this type of symptom including dairy, grains, nuts, gluten and GMOs. It may also be a sign that you are eating too much sugar and simple carbohydrates which include white flour and rice products. When you do not eat enough fiber or take supplements to help with digestion, it can cause gas, bloating and abdominal pain.

4. You find that you feel anxious or depressed for no reason

The presence of toxins in the blood affects neurotransmitters which are normally responsible for stabilizing moods. When the body is full of harmful substances that are released into your bloodstream, it can be difficult to have a positive outlook on life. People that are unable to detoxify properly may also have hormone imbalances which can cause symptoms such as breast tenderness, hair loss and even headaches.

5. You are suffering from fatigue

Fatigue is the result of a build-up of toxins in the body. When you don't have enough energy to get through the day, it can be frustrating. This can be due to things like chemical sensitivity, lack of sleep, poor diet and not drinking water throughout the day.

6. You get frequent headaches and/or back pain

Many people experience headaches on a regular basis but do not know how to cure them naturally. By eating more whole foods that are rich in vitamins and minerals, you will find that many problems such as headaches will go away after detoxing your body for a few days straight.

7. Your gums are inflamed

When you eat a lot of processed foods and sugar, it can cause an inflammatory condition in your body. This can lead to problems such as gum inflammation or bleeding as well as swelling which is known as gingivitis.

When you do not do a fast at least once a year, it can lead to bad bacteria growing in the mouth which could be contributing to the inflammation. If this is the case, adding in some foods that have anti-inflammatory properties like 1 tsp of raw apple cider vinegar and 1/2 tsp sage into your diet will help nourish your gums and teeth.

8. Multiple chronic health conditions are present

Your body produces toxins every day and if they are not regularly cleansed out, you will eventually get ill with some kind of infection or medical condition. The list of possible symptoms that can show up due to the build-up of toxins is long. When you do a fast, you will eliminate the imbalances in your body and allow your body to heal itself naturally.

CHAPTER 9: TURBOCHARGING INTERMITTENT FASTING

Intermittent fasting is potent. It is one of the key pieces I recommend for women over 50 years old. But it is not enough to maximize the metabolic potential in risk-prone individuals. In order to turbocharge intermittent fasting, you need to combine it with a healthy diet that extends beyond just food—think of balance (calories in – calories out), sleep (quality and quantity), and activity frequency.

Intermittent fasting and exercise working together

Think of it as a very powerful medicine for women over 50 years old. It's like a herbal supplement mixed in with the famed Slim-Fast shakes and then topped off with jogging. People who begin intermittent fasting lose more fat than those who only do regular exercise. This is because intermittent fasting activates your body to make new cells that burn fat. That means immediately after you had food, your body uses the time before and during the fast to repair cells and make more of them. After that, it can be converted into fat for fuel instead of muscle

The research on intermittent fasting is still relatively young. Early studies have been done on mice. One of the first studies in humans was conducted in Germany. These researchers found that women who followed a calorie-restricted intermittent fasting diet lost more weight than women who only did regular exercise. However, our bodies cannot be fooled by intermittent fasting for long periods of time. You will still need to continue eating enough in order to prevent malnutrition, but you will not be able to maintain the fasts' effects on your metabolism if you do not make some adjustments to your diet with exercise. Exercise can also help you achieve more because it burns energy that is stored as fat.

INTERVAL TRAINING

Interval training is one of the best ways to get the most out of intermittent fasting. You do not need to exercise for several hours a day to burn your fat stores. Intermittent fasting has more impact on your metabolism because when you exercise, you are also burning fat as fuel and then repairing cells at night so that your body can make more cells that burn fat. Everyone, including women over 50 years old, should do at least 30 minutes of interval training per week.

It's easier than you think—like burst training. Burst training is interval training with very short bursts of high-intensity exercise and longer periods of low-intensity activity. It is great for women over 50 years old because when you exercise, your body burns off energy stores. Fortunately, when your body is deprived of carbohydrate fuel during the fast and when you exercise, the energy that is used to fix your muscles and organs comes from fat instead of muscle.

Burst training is a good way to shed those extra pounds because it burns off more calories than aerobic training while using less time. You can burn about 400 calories in 30 minutes by doing burst training three times per week. But the reason I recommend burst training to women over 50 years old is that it also helps them reduce their belly fat, which most women tend to gain after menopause as they lose muscle mass and estrogen levels decline.

<u>Why you should exercise while intermittent fasting</u>

1. For added weight loss

Exercise and intermittent fasting work together to make your body produce more fat-burning cells. Doing both together also puts you in a great position to reduce belly fat and to lose weight.

Exercise also helps increase the levels of leptin, which is a hormone that signals how full you are. This means that if you exercise while intermittent fasting, you can eat more without feeling hungry or gaining weight. Exercise also helps boost your insulin sensitivity, which is the ability of your cells to use glucose for fuel instead of storing it as fat. You will turn those extra pounds into muscle instead of fat because exercise helps your body use the energy it needs for growth and repair instead of storing it as fat.

2. For better health

Exercise helps prevent cardiovascular diseases because it improves your blood flow and normalizes high blood pressure. It also reduces stress and depression, which both make your body hold onto fat stores. Exercise can also help you sleep better at night. You will not only gain muscle mass while you exercise, but you will also have more energy to do things during the day. Plus, if you exercise regularly while intermittent fasting, you will burn fat even during rest periods, which means that your metabolism is always active and burning off calories wherever possible. This slows down the aging process as well as making your body more resilient to disease and fat gain from overeating in the future.

3. For better cognitive function

Exercise also helps to clear your mind so that you will not have as many distractions from food, which can influence your appetite. Since exercise improves your mood and mental clarity, it is a great way to stay focused while you are in the middle of an intermittent fast.

4. For better sleep quality during fasting

Interval training is a great way to burn fat and improve sleep quality during fasting. Interval training targets more than just your muscles and burns more calories than aerobic training because of the short bursts of high-intensity exercise and longer periods of low-intensity activity. It is also easier to recover from than aerobic exercise, which is much more wearisome.

If you want benefits for your heart and a better night's rest, try interval training exercises. This short burst of vigorous activity allows you to get in shape without having to worry about overexerting yourself. The best part is that you can do it all in a short period of time considering how much it increases your metabolism and fat-burning capacity.

What kind of interval training works?

Most fitness experts recommend doing 15 rounds of between 30 seconds and 2 minutes on high-intensity sprints with only 1 minute to catch your breath in between rounds. You should do this 3 times per week to get the benefits of exercise and intermittent fasting. You should also try to mix up your exercise routine by alternating between burst and steady-state training. If you prefer, you can also do 2-minute bursts with 1-minute rest periods.

Some of the best exercises for interval training include running, hill sprints, sprints in place, skipping rope, boxing, kettlebell swings or even jumping rope.

Calorie restriction in addition to intermittent fasting

Women over 50 years old who follow a calorie-restricted diet are better protected from age-related diseases. Calorie restriction is a way of eating that can extend your lifespan by up to 15–20 percent. On the other hand, those who eat more calories tend to have less muscle mass and bigger bellies. In contrast, you should practice intermittent fasting combined with calorie restriction because it is more effective in preventing disease than when you restrict your calories alone. One study found that intermittent fasting and a calorie-restricted diet had similar effects on glucose levels, fat mass, inflammation, and blood pressure compared to when women ate their regular diets.

Calorie restriction helps reduce inflammation because it helps us eat foods that are low in fat. As a result, our bodies burn less of our own fatty acids and more carbohydrate fuel when they are needed by our cells. That leads to less generation of free radicals that can damage cells, which eventually causes disease. Also, calorie restriction is associated with lower levels of blood glucose. The reason for the reduction in blood glucose is also related to free radical production since high blood sugar levels increase oxidization of molecules including fats, protein, and DNA. Calorie restriction can also make it easier to prevent obesity because women who eat fewer calories are more likely to absorb food correctly into their cells well and not store it as fat. This is because their gastrointestinal system is more sensitive to the effects of energy—which helps them absorb amino acids—than it is to the effects of calories. Calorie restriction also helps reduce glucose levels and prevent muscle protein breakdown. This is one purpose for which our cells use glucose, so a calorie-restricted diet can help us live longer and be more efficient at using glucose as fuel.

Calorie restriction is also especially important in preventing chronic diseases such as cancer and diabetes. A lot of times when we think of cancer, we think about tumors, but they can be found in other areas as well including blood vessels, lungs, liver, soft tissue and bone marrow. People die of cancer not necessarily because they have cancer (though that is part of the story) but because their bodies go into a state of chronic stress. Our cells need energy to function, and when our cells are in a state of chronic stress, we are not able to respond appropriately to the damage that is going on in our body. Chronic inflammation takes a lot of energy, so cancer and other diseases tend to be linked with chronic inflammation. The only way to prevent chronic disease is by reducing the amount of energy we take in through food, which means targeting calories.

So why focus on calories? Because that's the only real thing you can change about yourself, and it's really easy. Calories are everywhere—they are in the grains and beans you eat, in the milk and eggs you use, and even in the fruits and vegetables. The only things that you cannot get calories from are fats, proteins, and fiber. What's more, since they are so pervasive throughout your food supply, it is very easy for calorie-restricted women over 50 years old to get enough calories.

Why you should combine calorie restriction with intermittent fasting

1. It lowers the risk of contracting age-related ailments

Research has shown that when you do intermittent fasting and calorie restriction, you can achieve a long lifespan, but that is not the only benefit. Intermittent fasting and calorie restriction is also associated with lower risk for age-related diseases including heart disease and cancer. First of all, keeping your body in a constant state of hunger allows it to burn off more fat than when you are regularly eating. Calorie restriction also forces your body to use sugar as fuel instead of less efficient fat cells because if it doesn't get enough glucose (sugar) it will break down its own muscle cells for fuel.

Start intermittent fasting and calorie restriction to reduce your risk of heart disease. In addition, it is very important to keep your blood pressure under control because it can lead to heart disease and hypertension. Intermittent fasting helps reduce blood pressure because when you are in a fasted state, you will lose a lot of excess salt—which makes up about 20 percent of our body weight—along with water weight and fat mass. So if you combine calorie restriction with intermittent fasting, you will be less likely to suffer from chronic diseases later in life.

2. It helps prevent cancer

The major cause of cancer is inflammation caused by free radicals that collect around the body along with damaged cells instead of dying off rapidly after they cause tissue damage. The best way to avoid this by eating foods that reduce inflammation. Women over 50 years old who do intermittent fasting and calorie restriction are also less likely to suffer from chronic inflammation.

You can also reduce your risk of cancer by getting lots of fiber from foods like fruits, vegetables, beans, and grains and eating very few animal proteins and fats.

3. It helps prevent diabetes

People with diabetes have a lot of excess sugar in their blood because an enzyme is missing that normally converts glucose into energy for the body but cannot do so in the case of type 1 diabetes because it cannot produce insulin. On the other hand, people with type 2 diabetes convert glucose into energy too efficiently, and the body fails to respond to insulin in order to use it effectively.

There are many ways for women over 50 years old to prevent diabetes—intermittent fasting and calorie restriction is just one of them. You can also try eating foods that are less processed instead of fast food and processed food. Fruits, vegetables, yogurt, and grains are all good examples of this.

4. It reduces your risk for Alzheimer's disease

Inflammation increases the production of free radicals that cause damage to the brain. Free radicals make proteins out of their own amino acids, which means that they won't fold properly and they create protein strands that are very unstable, which means that it is an easy place for harmful proteins to get in and cause damage. This is why maintaining a healthy balance between oxygen supply and waste removal can help prevent dementia. When your body is exposed to free radicals, it tries to protect itself by reducing blood flow to the brain as well as making new blood vessels grow inside the brain. However, if blood vessels form in the wrong place or form too many blood vessels, they can cause inflammation. Epileptic seizures, migraines, and Alzheimer's disease are all associated with inflammation.

Since you are likely to be less susceptible to Alzheimer's disease as you get older, aerobic exercise is the best way to maintain brain health and reduce your risk of Alzheimer's disease. The type of stroke that occurs as a result of heart attacks and cardiovascular diseases also increases your risk of developing Alzheimer's disease later in life. Exercise reduces blood pressure and heart rate, which prevent blood vessels from forming inside the brain. Instead of trying to turn your brain off, you should try to prevent free radicals from damaging it.

5. It helps you live longer and have more energy

Women over 50 years old who follow an intermittent fasting plan with calorie restriction are better able to metabolize fats. In addition, calorie restriction helps prevent obesity because it makes women put on weight more slowly, so they can be more efficient at using calories as a fuel source for their cells instead of storing them as fat in their bodies.

The benefits of calorie restriction are not just due to the amount of calories you take in but also because it helps you resist disease caused by too much of something else. When you consume foods that cause too many caloric intake, your body makes a lot of fat and proteins to help you store those excess calories. However, if you don't have enough energy, your body will burn these extra calories and won't make as much energy as it needs in order to keep up with its basic functions such as breathing and brain function.

How to combine calorie restriction with intermittent fasting

There are only so many things you can do in a day, so the way to get the most out of intermittent fasting and calorie restriction is to combine them with more regular exercise. Calorie restriction is an important component of intermittent fasting because it provides women over 50 years old with a way to save up nutrition for the times when they can eat normally.

First thing that you need to do is find out how much calories you should be eating each day in order to lose weight as efficiently as possible. Women over 50 years old who follow intermittent fasting and calorie restriction should keep track of their calories by using a diet app that tells you exactly how many calories are in each food item and portion size.

There are many ways you can use intermittent fasting and calorie restriction to meet your goals. You need to make sure that you don't go over your daily calorie limit at any time of the day because it is not healthy for your body. First thing in the morning, eat a protein-rich breakfast—ideally you will follow this with a low-carbohydrate lunch as well—and skip dinner. In addition, try drinking 12–24 ounces of water two hours prior to lunch and dinner to help reduce your appetite.

Alternatively, you can eat a big meal at the start of the day, and try to eat less as the day goes on. You should definitely do this if you have a big lunch or dinner so that you don't feel hungry when you go to bed. In addition, if you notice that you are losing weight very slowly, then it might be a good idea to exercise more while following this diet to make up for any extra calories that aren't being burned off by your body.

A lot of people who practice intermittent fasting see amazing results in losing weight by eating one meal per day and eating high-quality protein and fat in lower quantities than they normally would throughout the rest of the day.

<u>Combining intermittent fasting with carb cycling</u>

Carb cycling is a way to make your body more efficient at metabolizing and using carbohydrates because it prevents you from getting too much of something, which means that your cells are not overworked. You can also benefit from carb cycling if you have a condition like metabolic syndrome—a condition in which diabetes and heart disease are combined—because it makes your body more resistant to insulin.

Carbohydrate metabolism is deregulated in patients with type 2 diabetes, so the best way to reduce insulin resistance while improving overall health is by eating a diet that is higher in protein like intermittent fasting and calorie restriction. The benefits of carb cycling include building lean muscle mass and boosting blood glucose levels after exercise in order to recover quickly.

When you follow a carb cycling plan, you eat carbohydrates in the form of fruits and vegetables, which are rich in antioxidants—nutrients that neutralize free radicals. You can also eat whole grains and legumes because of their high-fiber content, which is important for long term health. Carb cycling has been shown to reduce hunger and improve the function of mitochondria, which means that your cells can produce more energy with less effort. It also helps the body break down fat into ketones so that it is easier to burn as fuel instead of storing it in our bodies.

The best way to combine carb cycling with intermittent fasting and calorie restriction is to eat a low-carbohydrate breakfast to keep your hunger at bay for several hours, then eat high-carbohydrate foods like fruit or vegetables for your second meal. The third meal of the day should be the largest meal, which means that you should eat a lot of protein, and only have enough carbohydrates to get through the rest of the day.

Combining calorie restriction with fasting every other day

Many women over 50 years old have trouble losing weight because their bodies start burning fat more slowly. However, intermittent fasting allows women over 50 years old to control blood sugar levels and insulin sensitivity by helping them lose body fat faster than they would otherwise.

When you follow an intermittent fasting program, your body will go into ketosis, which is a state where it cannot get enough glucose to produce energy properly. When it is in this state, ketones are produced by the liver and released into the blood stream while fat stores are broken down to generate energy. The best way to make sure that you don't have too much fat in your body is to combine calorie restriction with fasting every other day. That way you can have more time between meals when your body is burning fat as fuel instead of storing it in its tissues.

Women over 50 years old who combine intermittent fasting and calorie restriction may find that it is easier for them to lose fat in the short term than if they were following an intermittent fasting program on its own. Use this fad diet only if you are not trying to lose weight but rather eating fewer calories than you need so that your body has the energy it needs to function properly. When you combine intermittent fasting with calorie restriction, it is important to eat a diet that is high in lean protein, low-carbohydrate, and vegetables and fruits because these are the foods that can help you stay full throughout the day.

<u>Why you should combine intermittent fasting with calorie restriction</u>

1. It helps your body fight free radicals

Free radicals are produced by the bodies as waste products that damage tissues instead of dying off quickly after causing tissue damage. Combining intermittent fasting with calorie restriction will help prevent cancer by reducing the levels of free radicals around the body along with damaged cells.

2. It helps reduce your risk for type 2 diabetes

Women over 50 years old who follow intermittent fasting and calorie restriction are able to better metabolize fats because of their decreased risk of obesity and insulin resistance. In addition, they are also more efficient at the use of calories as a source of fuel for their cells instead of storing them in their bodies as fat.

3. It reduces your risk for cancer and cardiovascular diseases

Excess weight increases inflammation, which is essential to avoid so that you don't get cancer or heart disease later in life. Inflammation is stimulated by consuming too many free-radicals in food that damage tissues instead of dying quickly after causing tissue damage. Intermittent fasting and calorie restriction reduce inflammation by helping your body fight free radicals.

4. It reduces your risk of Alzheimer's disease

The fat deposits in the brain associated with Alzheimer's disease make your neurons more susceptible to damage. Intermittent fasting and calorie restriction also help fight Parkinson's disease, Huntington's disease, and other neurodegenerative disorders that cause behavioural changes due to a loss or damage to certain brain cells. Intermittent fasting is especially important for women over 50 years old because it has been linked to better memory function and a lower risk of developing dementia. In addition, studies have shown that calorie restriction can help improve memory functions in animals.

5. It increases your lifespan

The longer you live, the longer your cells have to divide and repair themselves. That means that you are more likely to live healthier as well as be in a better position to avoid dangerous diseases when you are older. Calorie restriction has been associated with lower rates of cancer and diabetes because it helps control aging by slowing down the rate at which cells divide. Intermittent fasting also helps increase longevity because it dramatically reduces oxidative stress, which is caused by free-radicals that damage cells instead of dying off quickly after causing tissue damage.

6. It makes it easier to lose weight

Many women over 50 years old have trouble losing weight because their bodies get used to the same eating patterns. Intermittent fasting and calorie restriction can help your body get rid of fat more easily because it is changing its functions all of the time.

7. It helps you maintain a healthy weight by burning fat instead of storing it

The best way to lose fat is by focusing on building lean muscle mass, which causes your body to burn more calories even at rest in order to maintain muscle mass. Intermittent fasting and calorie restriction are also effective for reducing fat around your mid-section because they cause your body to burn more calories than it would otherwise. In addition, you should try to build muscle mass by exercising regularly in order to keep the fat off of your mid-section.

8. It helps you maintain a positive outlook on life

You will be able to think more clearly and be more positive about life if you stop worrying about how you are going to lose weight and start focusing on the things that you are doing right in life. Some studies have found that calorie restriction can help reduce the symptoms of depression, anxiety, and even traumatic brain injury.

9. It improves your memory by breaking down fat into ketones for burning as fuel instead of storing it in the body as fat

Intermittent fasting and calorie restriction help increase mitochondria activities in your body by allowing you to break down excess fat into ketones so that they can be used as fuel instead of being stored in your body as fat. Exercise also helps break down fat because it increases your activity level and causes you to burn more calories.

<u>How to combine intermittent fasting with calorie restriction</u>

1. Find out how many calories you can eat each day in order to lose weight as quickly as possible—anywhere from 1200–1500 calories are enough for most women over 50 years old to get started losing weight.

2. Eat a low-carbohydrate breakfast in the morning, and then eat two meals during the day that are high in vegetables and fruits since they have a lot of antioxidants and nutrients that can help reduce inflammation, which causes you to gain weight. In addition, make sure that your second meal of the day is high in lean protein because it will be harder for you to feel hungry between meals if you are eating protein every time you do eat food.

3. Eat a large meal that is lower in carbohydrates before going to bed so that you can have fewer calories during the rest of the day. You should also drink 12 to 24 ounces of water at least two hours before each meal to help reduce your appetite.

4. Instead of eating a lot of food for dinner, try eating a small amount of high-protein food and wait 20 minutes before eating more if you feel hungry again. That way you won't spend all night sitting around feeling hungry so that you are not getting enough sleep because your body is constantly trying to get fuel from food and failing.

5. Eat dessert slowly at night and drink coffee or tea throughout the day to help you avoid getting too hungry. Intermittent fasting and calorie restriction are better for your metabolism than calorie restriction on its own because they help burn more fat as fuel instead of storing it in your body as fat.

6. Try intermittent fasting for a week or two, then start eating low-carbohydrate meals like vegetables after you have lost three to five pounds because it is harder for your body to store fat if there isn't any other food stored around your midsection that you could gain weight from.

7. When you are watching your weight, there is no need to go hungry. You can combine intermittent fasting and calorie restriction with a diet that is high in fruits and vegetables, and low-carbohydrate foods that will help you feel fuller for longer periods of time so that you have less hunger pangs between meals.

8. Don't worry about what kind of exercise you should do besides walking to control your weight—this is the one thing that requires the least amount of effort to carry out.

<u>Combining intermittent fasting with Keto</u>

Many women over 50 years old have trouble losing weight because their bodies get used to the same eating patterns.

Intermittent fasting and calorie restriction can help your body get rid of fat more easily because it is changing its functions all of the time. Keto is a diet that allows you to eat as many calories as you want in a day, but forces your body to go into ketosis so that it can burn fat as fuel instead of storing it in your body as fat. In addition, keto helps you lose weight by making it more difficult for your body to store fat when there isn't any food around your midsection that could cause you to gain weight.

Benefits of combining intermittent fasting with Keto

1. You consume fewer calories

It helps you eat fewer calories because of the ketone changes that occur in the body when you are on a keto diet. Without enough carbohydrates to use for energy, your body has to take the fat that is stored around your midsection and turn it into a usable form of energy instead of storing it as fat. This ability to burn fat as fuel instead of storing it is one reason why women over 50 years old should combine intermittent fasting with Keto so they won't have to go hungry between meals while trying to lose weight.

2. You lose weight quickly

The keto diet helps your cells convert fat into energy more efficiently. In addition, the absence of carbs that cause you to store weight makes it easier for you to burn fat as fuel instead of storing it in your body as fat. You also burn some fat while you are sleeping because your muscles need energy while you are sleeping so they don't get hangry.

3. Fasting is not as tough on your body

Keto is a very healthy diet that will help keep your metabolism steady because of the removal of those unhealthy fats from around your midsection. Instead of having all of those fat storage organs in your body, your body will be burning energy from the fat that is stored in your cells and being used for fuel instead.

4. It improves your memory by breaking down fat into ketones for burning as fuel instead of storing it in the body as fat

When you are on a keto diet, you can burn more energy from the fats stored around your midsection than if you were on a low-carbohydrate diet without Keto because it is difficult for your body to store excess fat when there isn't any food around to use the excess as fuel. You will also have more energy to help you lose weight because your cells have the ability to burn fat as fuel instead of storing it in the body as fat.

5. You don't feel hungry and tired all day as much as you did before

Some studies have found that women over 50 years old who are able to go without eating for longer periods of time are more likely to lose as much weight quickly because they don't eat enough calories to make them hungrier between meals. With intermittent fasting, you can eat exactly the right amount of food so that you don't get hungry and spend all day feeling hungry.

6. You don't have to count your calories

You will be able to eat as much food as you want without worrying about overeating because of the calorie-in/calorie-out concept that is done in the keto diet. You can eat whatever you want and still lose weight because you will not be adding any additional calories to your diet.

7. You can eat whatever you like without gaining weight

Low-carbohydrate diets are often criticized and considered unhealthy because it is difficult for many people over 50 years old to limit their carbohydrate intake in order to burn more fat instead of storing it in their body as fat. The keto diet doesn't require any calorie counting or special recipes because you are allowed to eat whatever you want as long as it is low in carbohydrates.

8. It helps your cells burn carbs better so that you have more energy throughout the day

Your body has to burn its own fat for energy instead of using carbohydrates from the food that you eat when you are on a keto diet. Your cells become more efficient at burning fuel if they aren't used to relying on external sources of energy all of the time.

9. You can eat a lot of food without gaining weight

Many people over 50 years old are afraid that they cannot eat a lot of food on a keto diet because they believe that they will gain too much weight. Obesity is not caused by eating too many calories but by eating too many unhealthy fats, trans fats, high-carbohydrate foods, and sugary foods that cause insulin resistance as well as leptin resistance. The keto diet allows you to eat a lot of food without gaining weight because it causes your body to burn fat rather than storing it in the body as fat.

How to combine intermittent fasting with Keto

Knowledge is power. The more you know about different exercisers and lifestyle changes, the more it can help you to find the one that suits you best. Both intermittent fasting and keto dieting offer benefits for women over 50, but they are also very different in how they work. Intermittent fasting, for example, is a fast-forwarding technology that doesn't require calorie restriction while keto dieting does. In this article, we will learn how they can be combined to produce better results.

Although the term intermittent is often used synonymously with eating and fasting, we clarify that intermittent fasting is a technology that involves a specific type of diet. Adopting this technology not only helps you lose weight, but also boosts your metabolism and creates changes in your body after the break, allowing you to have a better control over your appetite and food cravings. In addition to losing excess weight, this kind of lifestyle change reduces the risk for cardiovascular diseases and helps you stay healthy in general during later years.

While a keto diet focuses on fat consumption as the major calorie source, intermittent fasting also requires a significant reduction in caloric intake. This is usually achieved by not eating for several days each week and by having one day of very low, moderate or normal calorific intake. For most women over 50 years old, eating fewer than 1,200 calories per day is recommended. In fact, most experts recommend that you lower your caloric intake to around 1,000 calories per day to maintain weight loss while using intermittent fasting for weight loss.

Many women over 50 years old who are trying to lose weight may feel that they have lost the willpower to keep a very small diet. In fact, this is a common problem because many of us can eat so much without even noticing it. For example, if you eat a sandwich in the morning for lunch, you will eat half of it between one course and another and then also take cappuccino or something. In this case, intermittent fasting is less likely to be effective for women over 50 years old.

Intermittent fasting and keto dieting – Two lifestyles, two weights to lose

The intermittent fasting and the keto diet are two of the most effective ways to lose weight. However, they may also seem like two very different approaches to health. They are different, but they can be used together. Any weight loss method, either intermittent fasting or keto dieting will help you reduce your weight if you use it consistently but with little or no change in how you live your life. The reduction of your caloric intake will also have a significant effect on your cholesterol levels and blood pressure as well as on normalizing the hormonal balance in your body.

This is not possible to achieve with a keto diet alone because it simply forces you to eat fat. In contrast, when using intermittent fasting, you will minimize the consumption of certain types of fat while increasing the use of certain other types. In addition to keeping your body in perfect balance and health, this will also help you maintain your energy throughout the day so that you can continue doing everything you normally do. You may have already noticed that many women are better than men at doing everyday activities because they have a better energy level and so they are able to live activities without feeling fatigue or exhaustion.

The intermittent fasting and keto diet are two excellent weight loss methods that can be used together, but you may have to make certain changes to them so that they achieve the best results.

A keto diet is usually very effective when you use it for fast results but if it is used alone, it may not be so good because the body takes a long time to adjust. When intermittent fasting is combined with a keto dieting, the results are usually better because we get fast benefits combined with sustainable benefits. For example, when you use a continuous feeding system with a fat burner in your meals, then you get the best of both worlds. The fat burning capacity is increased with the use of intermittent fasting and you can also use keto to keep your metabolism high.

CONCLUSION: PUTTING IT ALL TOGETHER

Intermittent fasting for women over 50 years can be very beneficial. Intermittent fasting, coupled with regular exercise, is a way to lose weight and maintain a healthier lifestyle. There are many benefits associated with intermittent fasting for women over 50 years, including lower risks for heart disease and diabetes which can lead to an improved quality of life. It is not only healthy but also safe as long as it is done under proper medical guidance and supervision. With all the positive effects intermittent fasting can have on an individual's health, it's no wonder this trend has become increasingly popular in recent years.

In this book, you have learnt about an intermittent fasting protocol that can be very beneficial for women over 50 years. It is not only healthy but also safe as long as it is done under proper medical guidance and supervision. As you have seen, the intermittent fasting protocol gives you the benefits of eating less while still maintaining a healthy lifestyle. The best part about this protocol is that it actually has numerous benefits and may yield a better result than 'traditional' diets for women over 50 years who are seeking to lose weight, maintain health and live longer.

There are many such protocols that can be used for weight loss, but not all have the same benefits or the same safety measures like this one. It is important to have a balance between maintaining a healthy body and diet, as well as making sure you get the recommended amount of food. Therefore, as long as the intermittent fast is done under proper medical supervision and guidance, the risk of developing health problems like gallbladder diseases or heart disease are much lower. The intermittent fasting protocol can be incorporated into your lifestyle very easily regardless of your age, which makes it an excellent way to lose weight and maintain overall health at the same time.

What's next

It's now time to implement what you've read in this book. This book is not just a self-help book. It is more than that. It's a book that teaches you HOW to achieve your dream lifestyle, the way you want it. And this lifestyle includes a healthy body and weight loss. So, implementing what you've read is the last part.

But even after implementing what you've read in this book, there are many things that need to be done. You need to go through the process of 'learning by doing'. That means practicing the steps or decisions in this book until they become habit. It has been emphasized over and over again in this book that setting up your mind is very important.

This is also the process of 'building a good habit'. And in order to build a good habit, you need to start small. You need to start slowly, and then gradually increase your progress. It's also important to tell yourself why you are doing what you're doing. For example:

"Because I'm losing weight and my health is improving, I'm going to lose more weight every week."

Although this statement is true, it doesn't make it easier for our brain to remember or think about this motivation. However, saying something like this can make you more accountable for your actions and keep you focused on what's really important – weight loss results.

Well, that's about it for this book.

A request

I need your help getting this book to more people who need to read it. If you like this book, and can spare just a few minutes of your time to rate and review my book on Amazon, I would greatly appreciate it. It takes just a few minutes.